EATING FOR

For the good times

Eating For Peak Performance

Rosemary Stanton

UNWIN
PAPERBACKS

LONDON SYDNEY WELLINGTON

First published in Australia by Allen & Unwin Pty Ltd in 1988

First published in paperback by Unwin paperbacks, an imprint of Unwin Hyman Limited, in 1988

Unwin Hyman Limited
15–17 Broadwick Street
London W1V 1FP

Allen & Unwin Australia Pty Ltd
8 Napier Street, North Sydney NSW 2059 Australia

Allen & Unwin New Zealand Limited with the Port Nicholson Press
60 Cambridge Terrace, Wellington, New Zealand

ISBN 0 04 320223 3

CIP Data

Stanton, Rosemary
    Eating for peak performance.
    1. Sportsmen. Sportswomen. Physical fitness.
    Effects of diet
    I. Title
    613.7'1

Set in 12/12pt Baskerville by Times Graphics, Singapore
Produced by SRM Production Services Sdn Bhd, Malaysia

Contents

Preface　*vi*

1　The Western diet: How conducive is it to health and exercise?　*1*

2　Fats: Where are they?　*13*

3　Salt: Why it causes problems　*26*

4　Sugar: How much is too much?　*38*

5　Complex carbohydrates: The joy of eating more　*52*

6　Dietary fibre: Are you getting enough?　*63*

7　Alcohol: How to handle it　*75*

8　Protein: Animal or vegetable?　*86*

9　Iron, calcium and other minerals　*97*

10　Vitamins: Food or pills?　*118*

11　Weight: How do you get it right?　*136*

12　Eating for peak performance in sport　*155*

13　Planning the day's meals　*173*

Appendixes　*191*

Index　*199*

Preface

MANY of the world's top athletes have discovered that their sporting performance is affected by what they eat. Runners, rowers, tennis players, triathletes, cyclists, footballers and even yachtsmen have increased their energy levels by altering their diet. They have discovered that healthy eating not only helps them to achieve peak performance in sport, but also makes them feel better. As a bonus, most have found that healthy foods taste great. Later in life, their arteries, kidneys, liver and other body organs will be grateful for having been rescued from the abuse of a poor diet.

Sportspeople have certainly proved that you can eat to achieve peak physical performance. But such benefits are not confined to elite athletes. Amateur sportspeople, those who jog for pleasure, occasional fun-runners, weekend tennis buffs and those who simply enjoy a brisk after-dinner stroll will find that they too can eat for peak physical performance.

And for those who are continually fighting the battle of the bulge, a healthy diet, usually with more, but better-quality food, means you can feel fitter and become slimmer. The food which helps you to achieve peak performance also keeps you slim.

It's never too late to make a few simple changes in your choice of foods. They are neither difficult nor unpleasant. Quite the contrary. Healthy and enjoyable eating make a great combination: tempting the taste buds while giving the body the ideal ingredients to perform at its peak.

1

The Western diet:
How conducive is it to health and exercise?

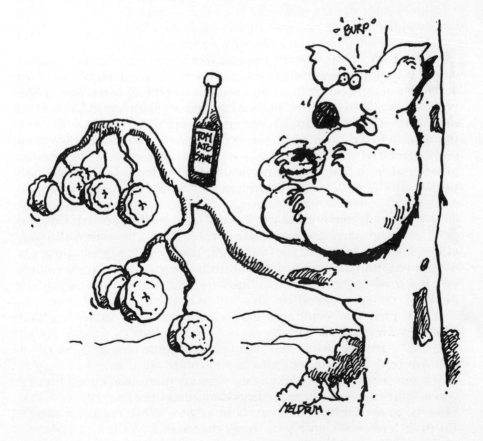

THE food supply available to the Western world is wonderful and varied. But, in spite of such abundance, many people fail to choose an adequate diet. In addition to all the healthy foods available, there has also been a proliferation of foods which are nutritionally useless. Advertising and promotions have guaranteed many of these foods a prominent role in the average daily diet. For the first time in human history, it is now possible to have a kitchen full of foods, but still miss out on those which are essential for the body to function at its full potential.

This does not mean that we need a magic vitamin pill or some other supplement. A poor diet cannot be fixed by a tablet or powder or special herbal mixture; in spite of the healthy bank balances of those marketing them, a lack of vitamins is not a major nutritional problem in most developed countries. Our major dietary problems are due to poor choice of foods. It is time to look at the nutritional quality of the foods we choose so that we can make healthier choices and gain the advantage and pleasure of healthy bodies.

With all the great-tasting healthy foods available in abundance why do so many people make poor choices? It is partly because we have been taught so little about nutrition and the workings of the human body. It is also because we have been seduced by slick food advertisements for gimmick items. So keen are we to fill the supermarket trolley with the latest convenience foods that we tend to forget the wonderful fresh foods which have so much to offer in nutritional benefits, as well as taste. Fresh fruit is the ultimate convenience food but it tends to be forgotten when we are bombarded with promotions for highly processed foods. There are hundreds of advertisements for foods which are high in fat, salt and sugar but how many do you see for carrots or peaches or most fresh foods? The profit level from most unprocessed foods is not great enough to generate huge advertising campaigns and many growers have few marketing skills. Most 'junk foods', on the other hand, are relatively cheap to produce and are skilfully promoted. Increasingly, we purchase what food manufacturers want us to buy and forget the body's basic needs.

Over the past 50 years, our eating habits have changed. Some of these changes have been beneficial, but many have not. Looking at our current diet, we find that many people are making such poor food choices that it is not surprising that exercise is so often regarded as an unpleasant chore. The typical Western diet is totally unsuited to physical activity.

Like other Western countries with a plentiful food supply, we spend our money on products which are high in fat, salt and sugar and lacking in dietary fibre and the basic complex carbohydrate so essential for adequate energy stores within the muscle cells. Cereals, grains, fruits and vegetables are much more suitable for physical activity than highly refined, sweet, salty and fatty foods.

The dieter's problem

The typical weight-reduction diets appearing in books and magazines have even less of the carbohydrate so essential for physical activity. Bread, potatoes and grain foods, all excellent sources of complex carbohydrates, are generally regarded as diet no-no's. As explained in chapter 11, any diet which omits carbohydrate will cause an initial weight loss. This is due to a drop in the body's normal water content, a loss of glycogen in the muscles and some loss of lean muscle tissue itself. There is very little loss of fat. Seeking instant results, many people equate the initial reduction in body weight with success. In fact, the lost weight usually returns—often with a few bonus kilos. In the meantime, the loss of muscle glycogen makes exercise even more of an effort, while the loss of some of the body's lean muscle tissue results in the flabby and haggard look so common in some perpetual dieters.

The need for carbohydrate

It is carbohydrate which enables the muscle cells to function properly so that efficient exercise is possible. Conversely, a lack of carbohydrate makes exercise more difficult. Contrary to popular belief, taking extra vitamins will not give you added energy for exercise. The conversion of carbohydrate to energy requires vitamins but the very foods which supply complex carbohydrates are also rich in essential vitamins and minerals. Taking extra vitamins without the basic source of fuel, the carbohydrate, is useless.

The human body is basically a machine, undoubtedly the most wonderful piece of machinery ever conceived. But, like any piece of machinery, the body needs care. It must be:

- given the right fuel;
- provided with proper maintenance; and
- regularly put through its range of physical activities.

If you do not give your car fuel, oil and water, if you neglect to service it, or if you never get it out of first gear, you can hardly expect top performance. The body is similar: if its needs are ignored, if it is not given the care it requires, or if it is seldom used for the purposes for which it was designed, it will not function properly. Muscles which do not receive proper fuel and exercise will fail to perform. Before long, unused muscles disappear and expanding midriffs and multiple chins take over.

Muscle cells must be used and supplied with fuel, preferably complex carbohydrate. Sufficient water is also vital. Both these ingredients are lacking in the modern Western diet. Minerals, vitamins and the amino acids, which are the end-product from the digestion of protein, are also important but even they cannot make up for a lack of the basic ingredients: carbohydrate and water.

Ironically, many people fail to eat sufficient complex carbohydrate because it is cheap and totally ignore something as free as water. Instead, we buy expensive, highly processed foods and drinks, and top them off with even more costly supplements in an attempt to repair the damage. Sales of soft drinks, various highly processed 'junk' foods, vitamins, amino acids, various herbal supplements and even dietary fibre pills are at an all-time high, while the consumption of grains, potatoes and bread, the most basic complex carbohydrate foods, has fallen steadily since the 1940s. If we were to eat more wholemeal bread, grains, vegetables and fruits, there would be no need for most supplements

THE TYPICAL DIET

Too much fat

Our diet undoubtedly contains far too much fat for our health. Few people rush into the kitchen asking for some fat when they're hungry. Most people will not even admit to liking fat. Nevertheless, fat dominates our diet. Fat is found in so many foods that it has become difficult to avoid.

The high-fat level causes more health problems than any other aspect of our diet. Eating fat increases body fat simply because fats contribute more kilojoules than anything else. Too much dietary fat is also related to coronary heart disease, stroke, high blood pressure, diabetes, gallstones and certain types of cancer, especially of the bowel and hormone-dependent areas (breast, uterus and prostate).

Some fats are obvious. Oozing out of sausages, hanging off the edge of steak, dripping out of fried chicken, or in the form of butter, margarine and oil in the home kitchen; you can't miss them. But there are also fats which are impossible to see, even if you had thought of looking for them in the unlikely foods they inhabit.

Fat is added to toasted muesli, for example, and accounts for almost 40 per cent of its kilojoules. The carob bar, which most people assume makes a healthy snack, has 53 per cent of its kilojoules coming from fat: the same percentage as a meat pie. And a major brand of tofu icecream (the darling of the health food shops) has 45 per cent of its kilojoules coming from fat: about the same level as regular icecream.

And then there is fat marbled through meat and stuffed inside

4

sausages, saturating chicken skin and fast foods, emulsified in mayonnaises and dressings, and a major part of cream, cheeses and nuts. Heaps of fat also come via cakes, biscuits, pies and pastries, potato crisps and other crunchy snack foods. The trendy croissant is laden with fat, made even worse if you top it with butter.

So many of our foods contain fat that it now accounts for about 30–40 per cent of the kilojoules in the average diet. Some fat can be used by the body for energy and some fats contain fatty acids which are essential to keep cell membranes healthy. However, such fats are only needed in small quantities and occur in foods such as fish and other seafood, in game meats and very lean meat, in soya beans, wholegrains, seeds and nuts. None of these foods is 'fatty'; we do not need to eat any obviously fatty foods to satisfy the body's requirements for essential fatty acids. In fact, many obviously fatty foods lack the essential fatty acids.

Fatty foods dominate the diet to the extent that other, more nutritious foods tend to be 'crowded out'. For example, many people skip a good thick slice of healthy wholemeal toast at breakfast in favour of a fatty cream bun or a high-fat doughnut for morning tea. At lunch, a bag of hot chips too often takes the place of a hearty salad sandwich and sausages readily replace leaner meats at dinner.

Fatty food choices contribute far more kilojoules than the foods they replace and they usually have fewer nutrients. Low-fat foods are usually much richer in essential nutrients and contain more complex carbohydrate and dietary fibre.

Fat or fibre

With the exception of nuts, few foods contain both fat and fibre. Most high-fat foods are totally deficient in dietary fibre. Chocolates, pastries, biscuits, sausages, red meats, mayonnaise, cheese, butter, oils and margarine are all high in fat and have no dietary fibre. Because of this, some of these foods do not satisfy like fruits and wholemeal bread. Without sufficient fibre, it is easy to take in more kilojoules than the body needs, simply because the foods look small and you don't feel very full after eating them. For example, you could eat six large apples for the same kilojoules as a 100–gram bar of chocolate. Few people could eat so many apples in one sitting, but the fibreless fatty chocolate would go down quite easily. It is very easy to overconsume fatty foods which lack dietary fibre.

Too much sugar

The average intake of sugar in the Western world is enormous. It ranges from about 400 grams to over double that per day. If you eat less, someone else is eating your share as well as their own.

There's probably nothing wrong with eating small amounts of sugar. But health authorities all over the world are unanimous that quantities as great as those now consumed are excessive. Every country which has established dietary guidelines has called for a reduction in sugar intake. Such advice certainly applies in countries of the rich developed world.

Sugar cane comes complete with a full set of vitamins, minerals, amino acids and plenty of dietary fibre. During the processing to make the white crystals, every vestige of these nutrients is removed. The result is a food which is chemically pure, nutritionally useless and anything but natural. It is the complete lack of dietary fibre which makes sugar so easy to overconsume. If we had to chew the cane, there would be no way we could ever get through the enormous quantities which are now commonplace.

Sugar easily replaces other, more nutritious foods. It also makes fats more palatable. Few people would eat chocolate, cakes, biscuits, icecream, many desserts and confectionery items if sugar didn't make their fat so desirable. In this way, sugar assumes a double culprit role.

As a carbohydrate, sugar itself contains only as many kilojoules as the complex carbohydrates. But sugar has none of the essential nutrients which accompany the carbohydrate in foods such as fruits, vegetables, breads, cereals and grains. Nor is it filling. It's easy to eat or drink vast quantities of the stuff. A cup of tea with sugar, for example, is no more filling than one without. Similarly, a can of sugar-sweetened soft drink contains ten teaspoons of sugar, but provides no more satiety than a sugar-free drink. The contents of some breakfast cereals are almost half sugar. Some of this sugar replaces cereal fibre making highly sweetened cereals much less filling. Most people feel far less 'full' after a bowl of chocolate popped cereal than if they had eaten porridge or unsweetened, untoasted muesli.

The carbohydrate in sugar can certainly be used as a fuel by the muscles. However, sugar is an inferior food when compared with fruits, vegetables, cereals, breads and grains. There is no reason why those who are physically active should not include some sugar in their diet, as long as it does not replace foods of better nutritional quality and is not consumed within the hour prior to strenuous physical activity (see chapter 4).

With the average sugar intake contributing more than 400–500 kilojoules (1700–2100 Calories) a day, it is obvious to everyone, except the sugar industry, that sugar can contribute to excess weight. Some of this excess weight also comes from fats which sugar has made so palatable. Added to this is the harmful effect of sugar on teeth. With a population riddled with excess flab, it does not make sense to waste so much of our kilojoule intake on sugar.

Too much salt

For many years, salt enjoyed a high status. Since sweat contains salt, many people who were physically active enough to sweat profusely thought that they should eat extra salt. Others who lived in hot climates or worked in hot conditions thought that salt tablets were necessary to replace their losses (see chapter 3).

Salt is sodium chloride and we need both sodium and chloride. However, the average Western diet contains about ten times as much sodium as the body needs. Most of the excess comes from the high-salt content of many processed foods.

Those who sweat profusely need a little more sodium than others. However, the body is so good at conserving sodium that those who sweat regularly soon put out less sodium in sweat. Trained athletes who do not eat a lot of salt lose much less salt in their sweat than someone who is unaccustomed to physical activity. With heavy sweating, there is also less sodium than usual lost in the urine. A lack of salt is rarely a problem; an excess frequently is.

The high level of salt in the diet is responsible for high blood pressure, a problem which affects hundreds of thousands adults and an increasing number of children. Some people's bodies are more sensitive to a high salt intake than others, but we cannot yet predict who is likely to suffer harmful effects from salt and who will not. Since no healthy person needs so much salt, it makes sense for everyone to discover the natural taste delights of foods without added salt. Processed foods with no added salt or a low-salt content can also be useful.

Too much alcohol

Assuming that those under 15 years of age do not indulge in alcohol, the rest of the population consumes a yearly average of over 100 litres of beer, about 11 per cent of it as low-alcohol beer. Added to that, the average person quaffs over 200 glasses of wine (about 115 millilitres) and around 5 litres of spirits. When you consider that some people do not drink alcohol, many people obviously have an even higher intake.

Such large quantities of alcohol provide many kilojoules which contribute to excess weight and its attendant health problems.

Alcohol in small quantities (one to two drinks a day) appears to do no harm to most people and may even be beneficial. Some studies have shown greater longevity in those who drink at this level compared with those who have no alcohol. Whether the alcohol contributes to longer life through its relaxant effects or has a direct effect on blood fats (and thus on heart disease) is not yet known. Early reports that alcohol increased the levels of a good type of cholesterol have since been amended (see chapter 2).

In moderate quantities, alcohol provides a relaxing effect which most people find pleasant. It does not stimulate the body, although it can remove inhibitions and increase some people's sociability. In larger quantities, alcohol causes health problems which are estimated to cost the community hundreds of millions a year.

The health problems include damage to the liver, brain, heart and pancreas. Since alcoholic drinks provide many kilojoules, alcohol is also responsible for much of the excess weight in the community, particularly among men (see chapter 7 for more details). Social behaviour also takes a downward slide in anyone who drinks too much and/or too often. And the final nail in the coffin relates to the well-established connection between alcohol and accidents, especially car accidents.

Women and alcohol

Alcohol affects women differently at particular times. At times it can be difficult to walk in a straight line after two or three glasses of wine, whereas, on other occasions this quantity of alcohol causes no obvious effects. Early reports that alcohol was absorbed faster into a woman's blood at different times of the menstrual cycle have not been supported by later research. However, researchers have shown that alcohol has a much more intoxicating effect on most women just before the beginning of the menstrual cycle and for the first few days of the period.

Too little complex carbohydrate

The typical Western diet provides only a third to a half of the quantity of complex carbohydrate needed for peak performance.

Carbohydrate is the primary source of fuel for the body. Both fat and protein can be used to provide energy, but complex carbohydrate is the favourite source of energy for the muscle cells. Physical activity increases the demand for complex carbohydrate.

Complex carbohydrate foods are generally good sources of vitamins, minerals and dietary fibre. This further enhances their value over the simple carbohydrate found in sugar.

The major sources of complex carbohydrate were once bread and potatoes. Most people ate few grains apart from some rice, corn or the occasional bowl of rolled oats, and had seldom if ever tried rye, wheat, barley, sorghum, millet or buckwheat. Cereals foods were confined to a bowl of breakfast cereal and the occasional plate of spaghetti (generally swamped with a fatty meat sauce). In some countries legumes were not eaten, mainly because no—one knew how to cook them.

Over the past 40 years, the national diet has plunged even further into complex carbohydrate deficiency. Bread consumption has almost halved, fewer potatoes are eaten as potatoes (although potato crisp and chip consumption has increased dramatically), most grains are still not eaten, the bowl of breakfast cereal has become two–thirds of a bowl of cereal and one third of a bowl of sugar (in some cases, even more sugar), and many people still do not have a clue what to do with legumes. Only pasta consumption has risen.

There are two major factors working against increasing the consumption of complex carbohydrate foods:

1   Because most sources of complex carbohydrate are cheap, they are often regarded as 'fillers' or 'poor man's food'.
2   Most slimming diets published as books or magazine–newspaper articles have consistently preached the 'no carbohydrate' gospel.

A 'poor man's diet' is actually ideal for anyone who wants to use the body for physical activity. Peasants and others who live largely on complex carbohydrate are able to work hard all day because they are supplying the body's muscles with the favourite source of fuel for efficient performance. The adoption of high-protein but fatty foods has led to muscles being replaced with flabby midriffs, soft arms, sagging buttocks and multiple chins along with rolls of flesh around the waist. By despising 'filler' foods, we have filled our bellies with flab rather than providing muscles with food which enables them to stay firm and strong.

The argument that anyone wanting to lose weight should avoid carbohydrates doesn't hold water. In fact, when the diet is deficient in carbohydrate, the body loses a lot of water. It is this water loss which accounts for the temporary weight loss seen with low-carbohydrate diets. There is little effect on the body's fat levels. The resulting state of partial dehydration is also hazardous for anyone who wants to exercise, since muscle cells must have sufficient fluid to function efficiently.

Perhaps the final evidence that the low-carbohydrate slimming diets do not work is shown by the number of overweight people in the community. In the days when complex carbohydrate made up a much larger portion of the daily fare, the population was far slimmer. Admittedly, our grandparents had much more physical activity, but, then again, their diet provided the fuel to make this activity possible. Our modern-day diet, deficient in complex carbohydrate, is not conducive to physical activity.

Sportsmen and women have been discovering the benefits of increasing their intake of complex carbohydrates. Muscle cells can function longer, performance improves and energy levels are much

9

higher with more complex carbohydrate. The amount of energy stored in muscles in the form of glycogen (a storage form of carbohydrate) increases with more complex carbohydrate. Some increase can also be achieved with sugar, but the benefits are less in the long term. As discussed in chapter 4, sugar creates other problems.

Too little dietary fibre

Each year millions of doses of laxatives are sold. And that is not counting the fibre supplements, unprocessed bran and the various herbal and fruit mixtures sold in health food shops. We can safely assume that we are a constipated lot!

Constipation is caused by a lack of dietary fibre. Too little fluid can exacerbate the problem. The fact that we undervalue complex carbohydrate foods has led to a fibre deficiency since the cereals, grains, breads, vegetables and legumes which supply complex carbohydrate are also sources of dietary fibre. There has also been a tendency with the few carbohydrate foods that we do eat to process them to the extent that much of the fibre is lost. Cornflakes, for example, have almost no fibre, unlike the corn from which they were made. Fruits provide dietary fibre, but there is a tendency for fruit to be consumed more in the fibreless form of fruit juice than in their natural state.

Most nutrition authorities recommend a daily intake of at least 30 to 40 grams of dietary fibre. The average Western intake is less than half this amount.

Dietary fibre comes in a variety of forms and these have different actions within the body (see chapter 6). Recent research has shown that some types of fibre are valuable in helping to control blood sugar in diabetics and in those with fluctuating blood sugar levels. Blood cholesterol may also be controlled by certain types of fibre. However, research shows that it is important to eat the high-fibre foods, rather than trying to isolate the fibre and take it as a pill.

Foods which are rich in dietary fibre include vegetables, legumes, wholegrain cereals, wholemeal and wholegrain breads, and fruits. These foods also supply a wide range of vitamins and minerals and some are sources of protein. Dietary fibre only occurs in vegetable foods; animal products have none.

Dietary fibre is filling. Most people will not overeat foods which are rich in dietary fibre. Unfortunately, some people confuse 'filling' with 'fattening' and reject foods simply because they are filling. 'Filling' foods help control body weight since you are much more likely to stop eating when your stomach feels full.

Foods which have no dietary fibre slip down so effortlessly that the natural satiety mechanism does not come into play. Fruit juices,

10

for example, are much less filling than the fruits from which they are made. Most people would find it difficult to eat five apples, but relatively easy to consume their juice—and their kilojoules. So, while it would be difficult to gain weight by eating a high-fibre food like apples, the processed version makes overconsumption easier. A bowl of cooked rolled oats contains lots of fibre and is filling; a light-weight sugary cereal has the same number of kilojoules, but is much less filling so that you are more likely to eat other foods. Such logic has escaped many consumers who have assumed that they must not eat a food such as porridge, because it is filling, and therefore, fattening. Nothing could be further from the truth.

Eating for peak performance

Whatever your level of physical activity, the ideal diet is one which provides:

- a high level of complex carbohydrate and dietary fibre;
- plenty of water;
- little fat;
- sufficient, but not excessive, protein; and
- a source of calcium, iron, other minerals and vitamins.

Translated into foods, this means a daily intake consisting of:

1 Plenty of water.
   Quantity: as desired but at least 6 to 8 glasses a day. Some can be in the form of tea (preferably weak) or mineral or soda water. Athletes who train each day will need much more.
2 Plenty of vegetables, either as salads or steamed, stir–fried or microwaved.
   Quantity: as desired, but at least some salad and 3 to 4 different vegetables.
3 Fruit of any type.
   Quantity: as desired, but at least 2 to 3 pieces a day, preferably as whole fruit rather than as juice (some juice is fine).
4 Wholemeal or wholegrain bread or some white bread, rolls or muffins.
   Quantity: as desired, but at least 4 to 6 slices a day. Athletes will need 8 to 12 slices, or more.
5 Grains or cereal foods such as rolled oats, wholegrain break-fast cereals, rice, pasta, cracked wheat or any other grain.
   Quantity: as desired, but at least one serving.
6 Protein from foods such as fish or other seafoods, chicken, turkey or game, very lean meat, or an alternative such as eggs, dried beans, peas, lentils or tofu.

11

Quantity: one serve a day (75 to 100 grams of cooked meat or ¾ cup of beans; fish can be eaten in larger quantities). Larger quantities are suitable for those who are very active but should not replace bread, cereals and grains, fruits and vegetables.

7   Some dairy products, preferably low-fat or reduced-fat varieties. Low-fat yoghurt or cheese, preferably mozzarella, Swiss or other reduced-fat cheeses.

Quantity: 500 to 750 millilitres of milk (30 grams of cheese is equivalent to 150 millilitres of milk).

No matter what your level of physical activity, these basic dietary principles apply. The exact quantity of each type of food eaten depends largely on the individual. In general, the greater the degree of physical activity and the higher the content of muscle (as opposed to body fat), the more food required. Although there is some individual variation due to differences in basic metabolism, the energy requirements depend on the amount of physical activity and the level of lean body tissue. The more exercise you do, the greater the kilojoule requirements. And the higher the muscle content of the body, the greater the number of kilojoules needed. Since exercise produces muscle, those who are the most active usually need the most food.

Once body fat levels increase, it takes more kilojoules of energy to move the heavier body around. For some, the energy requirements for movement are so great that they develop an unconscious habit of not moving to any extent. This further reduces the muscle content of the body, since muscles which are not used are gradually lost.

The moral of this story is that the fat tend to become fatter while the lean have all the ingredients for remaining slim. The way to change from a fat to a lean person is to exercise and to eat foods which allow the body to exercise at its peak. Trying to exercise while following the typical Western diet (high in fat, sugar, salt and alcohol and low in the all-important complex carbohydrates and dietary fibre) is doomed to failure.

By switching to a healthier diet with more fruits, vegetables, breads, grains and cereals and with more seafoods and fewer fatty, sugary items, you will provide extra glycogen so that your muscle cells can begin to function at their peak. And don't forget the water.

2

Fats:
Where are they?

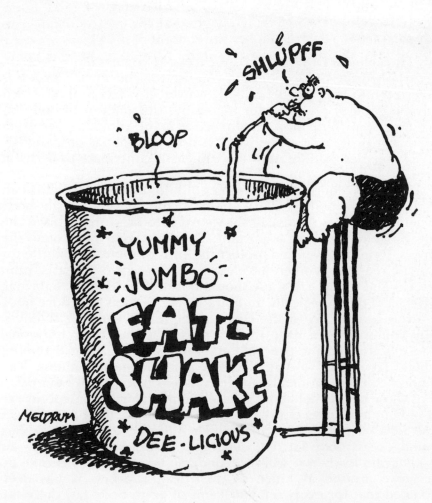

FEW people set out to eat a fatty diet, but fat is surprisingly tempting. It is the smell of fat wafting from a roast dinner that sets the taste buds tingling. It is fat which draws us, magnet-like, into a take-away food shop. And it is fat which we crave when we reach for a chocolate, a luscious-looking piece of cream cake, a pastry, croissant or a packet of crunchy savoury snacks.

It is also fat which clogs up the arteries, forcing the heart to work harder to push blood past the grease deposits. It is fat which makes life difficult for our livers and gallbladders. And it is fatty deposits which bulge over the belt, hang under the chin, obliterate the shape of our lean tissue and wobble when we walk.

Body fat

Body fat can arise from any sort of excess. If you eat more protein, fat, carbohydrate or alcohol than you use for energy, the excess is converted into body fat deposits. However, it is fats in food which have the greatest potential for increasing the amount of body fat since they contribute more than twice as many kilojoules per gram than either protein or carbohydrates do. Alcohol has only slightly fewer kilojoules than fat, so it too can easily contribute to body fat stores.

Fats are such concentrated sources of kilojoules that it is difficult for the average body to burn them all for energy. So the body efficiently converts the excess fat we eat into fat stores around the body. Some of these are important. You need some fat around the kidneys, some to cover and protect the ends of joints and a little for aesthetic reasons. Women have extra fat deposits on breasts, hips, buttocks and thighs and these should not be regarded as abnormal. In fact, it is physiologically undesirable for women to reduce body fat levels too far. With the current vogue for extreme slimness, many young women have so little body fat that their hormonal balance is affected and they no longer menstruate. A small amount of body fat is also wise as a reserve for unexpected illness. You cannot, however, rationalise obvious flab as being at all essential.

For those people not about to face a famine, large fat deposits are not only totally unnecessary but are a burden for the body. To get some idea of the extra effort which must be expended to cart around excess body fat, try walking up a hill carrying a 10– or 20–kilogram load. You will soon understand why heavy people do not move around as much as their leaner peers. It has been estimated that for every ten kilograms of extra body fat, there are some 29 kilometres of extra blood vessels through which blood must be pumped. With such an increased burden to bear, it is little wonder that overweight people have a shorter life expectancy. The

14

opposite extreme, with minimal fat stores, is also unhealthy. The human body is designed to have a small store of fat, but not too much.

Looking at the health risks associated with excess body fat, we find that those who have excess fat around the waist and upper body (the 'apple' distribution) have the greatest risks of heart disease, gallstones, diabetes and high blood pressure. Those with fat around the hips and thighs (the 'pear'-shaped body) have little increased risks of these health problems (see chapter 11 for a full discussion).

However, any type of excess fat increases the likelihood of wear and tear on joints and will make problems such as arthritis worse. With the exception of osteoporosis and tuberculosis (both of which are more common in the underweight), excess body fat is a health hazard.

Let's take a specific look at different types of fats in foods.

TYPES OF FATS

According to their chemical structure, fats are described as saturated, monounsaturated or polyunsaturated. Most foods contain a mixture of all three types of fats. In an egg, for example, of the major fats present, 38 per cent are saturated, 47 per cent are monounsaturated and 11 per cent are polyunsaturated. However, there is usually one type of fat which predominates in foods, and most foods are placed in a category according to their major type of fat. All types of fats contribute exactly the same number of kilojoules. Polyunsaturated margarine is thus just as fattening as butter.

Saturated fats

Saturated fats are the villains in causing high levels of cholesterol in the blood. Contrary to popular belief, however, saturated fats are *not* synonymous with animal fats. The greatest portion of saturated fats in the diet does not come from eating foods such as lean meat and milk but from the saturated fats which find their way into fried foods, fast foods, many processed foods, biscuits, pies, cakes, pastries, chocolate, coconut and palm oil (widely used in commercial frying), many margarines and some types of confectionery. Of course, animal foods such as fatty meats, sausages, salamis, bacon, some processed meats, cream, butter, most cheeses and full-cream dairy products also contribute a lot of saturated fat. If you avoid only the obvious animal fats in meats and dairy products, however, you can still consume a lot of saturated fats which are present, but not necessarily visible, in processed foods.

Polyunsaturated fats

Polyunsaturated fats are found in foods as diverse as seafoods, vegetable oils, polyunsaturated margarines and mayonnaises, and many nuts and seeds. Wild meats, game and very lean flesh have very little fat, but a high proportion of what they do possess is polyunsaturated.

Some years ago, it was noted that polyunsaturated fats could lower the level of cholesterol in the blood. Vegetable oils were suddenly regarded as 'healthy' and special polyunsaturated margarines flooded the market. Advertising capitalised on the healthy image and consumption rose dramatically. Then several long-term studies reported a flaw in the argument. Groups of people who changed to polyunsaturated fats certainly gained some protection from heart disease, but their overall death rate changed very little; more of them died from cancer. This was not taken to mean that the polyunsaturated fats caused cancer; it probably reflects the fact that if you don't die from heart disease your chances of dying from cancer are increased. Nevertheless, polyunsaturated oils and margarines lost some of their support as new evidence pointed to the *total amount of fat* causing damage to various systems within the body. Too much of any kind of fat is undesirable. So, if you have always disliked the flavour of polyunsaturated margarine, you should no longer feel compelled to eat the stuff. Before you rush for the better–tasting butter, however, remember that it is still fat and all fats should be eaten in very small quantities.

There is also the question of the type of polyunsaturated fat. Those in vegetable oils are different from the polyunsaturated fats found in fish and other seafoods. In the vegetable oils, a fat called linoleic acid predominates. It belongs to a class of polyunsaturated fats called omega–6 fatty acids. Fish contain some linoleic acid but also have other polyunsaturated fats, including two which are commonly called EPA and DHA (the full names are eicosapentaenoic acid and docosahexaenoic acid). These fats belong to a class called omega–3 fatty acids and appear to have several possible benefits (see page 22).

Some plants also contain an omega–3 fatty acid, known as alpha–linolenic acid, found in leaf membranes rather than in the seed oils used to produce vegetable oils and margarines. Perhaps we have chosen to eat the wrong part of the plant!

Polyunsaturated fats are certainly valuable. But, like most aspects of nutrition, too much of a good thing turns sour. Saturating the diet with margarine does not provide overall health benefits. However, by eating fish you can take in the valuable polyunsaturated fatty acids without bombarding your body with a huge amount of fat. Total fat intake thus is kept low while maximising the benefits.

Monounsaturated fats

Monounsaturated fats occur principally in olive oil, peanut oil and peanuts, and avocados. For many years, these fats were thought to be neutral in the cholesterol debate. This was somewhat strange in view of the fact that populations who consume most of their fat as olive oil, have little heart disease. More recent research has shown that monounsaturated fats can actually lower blood cholesterol levels to some extent. With polyunsaturated oils having fallen from favour, olive oil has achieved a new status. Populations which use olive oil not only have a low incidence of heart disease, but also less cancer. It is worth remembering, however, that the typical Italian diet, even with its olive oil, has only about 20 per cent of its kilojoules coming from fat.

It should also be noted that much of the olive oil consumed throughout the world is cold pressed and is poured over food rather than used for frying. Heating, either during the extraction of oil or in cooking, may destroy valuable constituents of the oil.

The avocado, another source of monounsaturated fat is also a source of vitamin E. Criticism of the avocado as being one of the few fruits or vegetables to contain fat should cease. Avocados certainly do not contain pre-formed cholesterol, and even the type of fat they contain is above suspicion. The major problem with avocados is that their superb flavour encourages some people to eat too many and thus increases their total fat intake.

CHOLESTEROL

The villain of the 1970s, cholesterol, slipped out of the limelight for a while. Cholesterol is a fatty, waxy substance which looks something like the wax which accumulates in your ears. It should not be considered abnormal or even undesirable since it has a vital role to play in making vitamin D and some of the body's hormones (including sex and adrenal hormones). Cholesterol is also found in nerve and brain tissue and is an essential part of the membranes which surround all body cells. In spite of its vital role, we do not need to eat cholesterol since the body is quite capable of making its own supplies. Most of the cholesterol in the body does not come from the pre-formed cholesterol in food, but is made within the body from saturated fats.

Problems arise when some people take far too much cholesterol and the excess accumulates in the arteries, especially the coronary arteries. These arteries are branching structures with a diameter of 17 about the size of a drinking straw. They carry blood to the heart muscle itself. If the quantity of cholesterol in the blood rises, some of the waxy fat is deposited with other substances around the inside of the arteries. This means that there is less room for the blood to pass through. As a consequence, the heart must pump much harder to force blood through the coronary arteries. To make matters worse, it will take only a small clot of blood to block a partially clogged artery and shut off the blood supply, causing a heart attack. To prevent fatty cholesterol deposits forming in the arteries, it is essential to prevent the levels of cholesterol in the blood from rising.

Cholesterol in the blood comes from two main sources:

1   Eating foods which contain cholesterol (pre–formed cholesterol). These are all animal foods and include brains, liver, kidneys, egg yolks, meat, milk, cheese, butter, cream, poultry, fish and other seafoods. There is no pre–formed cholesterol in vegetable foods. Contrary to popular belief, avocados do not contain cholesterol. The pre–formed cholesterol occurs in lean meats as well as fatty meats since it is part of the structure of the cells in the animal flesh. As we shall see later, pre–formed cholesterol is mainly a problem when the basic diet is high in fat.

2   Eating foods which contain saturated fats. These fats are turned into cholesterol within the body. Saturated fats are found in both animal and vegetable foods. Major dietary sources include most commercially fried foods, fast foods, fatty meats, some processed meats such as sausages and salamis, butter, cream, most margarines, 'solid' cooking oils, coconut and palm oil (used in some processed and commercially fried foods), pastries, biscuits, cakes, most cheeses and full-cream dairy products.

Of the two sources of blood cholesterol, the saturated fats are the worst. Foods which contain pre–formed cholesterol are generally only a problem if they, or the basic diet, are high in fat. Both fish and meat, for example, contain cholesterol, but fish has very little fat and so its cholesterol content does not increase blood cholesterol levels. With the exception of extremely lean meat, most cuts of meat have much more saturated fat than fish and seafoods. Looking at the total picture of pre–formed cholesterol plus saturated fats, fish is a much better choice than most meat meals. Serve the fish battered and fried, however, and all the advantages are lost since the fish has now acquired a high level of saturated fat. In addition, the small amount of fat which fish does contain can reduce the levels of cholesterol in the blood. Fish is thus a good choice.

When considering whether a food will increase your blood cholesterol level, look beyond its pre–formed cholesterol and note its saturated fat level. If it has a high content of both cholesterol and saturated fat, avoid it, at least most of the time.

Using this criterion, we find that blood cholesterol levels are unlikely to increase with seafoods (unless dipped in batter and fried), very lean meats and poultry (cooked without fat and with fat removed), and even eggs (if cooked and served without a source of fat). So grill your fish, select the leanest possible meat and then trim off any remaining fat, avoid frying meat or chicken, and boil, poach or scramble your egg rather than frying it in the saturated fat which comes out of bacon or butter.

Shellfish such as prawns, lobster and crab were once considered to be undesirable foods for anyone concerned about cholesterol. Early measurements of the cholesterol content of foods inadvertently included some other sterols which have since been found to have no adverse effect on blood cholesterol levels. Recent measurements show that lobster and crab have very little cholesterol. Squid and prawns have slightly higher levels but an average serving of either of these foods can still be included. Prawns, like all seafoods, have very little fat and their cholesterol level is no reason to damn them. However, avoid battered or fried prawns. Oysters, crab and lobster have very little fat or cholesterol and can be included as often as you please (or can afford!).

When most people eat a food containing cholesterol, such as an egg or some liver, the level of cholesterol in the blood does not necessarily increase. Eating a source of pre–formed cholesterol means that the body should not need to make its own cholesterol. Or you may simply excrete what you do not need. If you have a body which does not cut out its own cholesterol production when enough is being supplied in the diet, you should be somewhat wary of foods containing pre–formed cholesterol and especially vigilant in avoiding saturated fats. It is the saturated fats which have the greatest potential to increase levels of cholesterol in the blood. If you are carrying too much body fat, you are also more likely to have high levels of cholesterol in your blood.

HDL and LDL

To complicate the picture, there are different types of cholesterol. Since fats do not dissolve in the blood, they attach themselves to protein molecules which carry them around. These combined protein–fat molecules are called 'lipoproteins'. The two best known are HDL and LDL (high- and low-density lipoprotein). HDL is a 'good guy' 19 and picks up excess cholesterol from the arteries so that it can be excreted. HDL cholesterol is protective against heart disease and higher levels occur in athletes, those who are very lean, some young women, and people from long-lived families. LDL is the 'bad guy' and contributes to the fatty deposits which thicken the walls of the arteries. Men tend to have higher levels of LDL than young women. After menopause, there is little difference between levels of LDL in men and women.

To some extent, your HDL and LDL levels are predetermined by heredity. However, you can increase your HDL levels with exercise and by staying slim. If you are a young, lean female athlete whose relatives lived to a ripe old age, it is highly likely that your HDL levels are high. If you are older, overweight and largely sedentary, and your family tree has few octagenarians, you will need to make an effort to lose weight, exercise more and so increase your levels of the beneficial HDL cholesterol.

Alcohol in small quantities is sometimes thought to increase HDL, but recent research has shown that it is more likely to increase one of the other forms of cholesterol. Further research is needed to help us to understand their roles.

A blood test can determine your levels of cholesterol. Ideally, you should have your HDL and LDL levels measured since it is now considered that the ratio of these is more important than the actual level. Most people whose total cholesterol level is high find they have high levels of the nasty LDL. The recommended maximum total cholesterol level is 5.5 millimoles per litre (210mg/100ml in the old measurements). This has recently been reduced from the previous recommendation of 6.5 millimoles per litre because it was found that the new 5.5 level represented a lower risk of heart disease. HDL cholesterol usually makes up 20 to 30 per cent of the total cholesterol. Some marathon runners have been found to have up to 50 per cent of their cholesterol in the protective HDL form. The higher the proportion of HDL, the better.

Effect of dietary fibre

Certain types of dietary fibre can reduce blood cholesterol levels. About half of the cholesterol made in the body is converted to substances called bile salts which help us to digest fats. Once a meal is over, the bile salts are reabsorbed into the blood and recirculated for further use. Certain kinds of dietary fibre remove these bile salts from the blood. This means that more cholesterol is converted into bile salts and the level of cholesterol in the blood is lowered. The kinds of dietary fibre which have this property are pectin and

saponins. Pectin is found in fruits while saponins occur in soya
beans, alfalfa, mung beans and sprouts, other dried beans, peas,
peanuts, spinach, asparagus and oats.

Recent studies suggest that acids produced during the fermentation of the gummy types of fibre in oats and legumes may also
lower cholesterol (see chapter 7). These foods are beneficial for
those with a high cholesterol level. The type of dietary fibre in
unprocessed bran and most cereal fibres does not work in this way.

Lecithin

This substance belongs to a group of phospholipids, which are
compounds of phosphorus and various fatty acids. Lecithin also
contains a substance called choline. In spite of the great claims made
for it when sold as a 'health food' supplement, lecithin occurs widely
in both plant and animal foods and is also one of the most commonly
used emulsifiers in processed foods. (Emulsifiers help keep fat
evenly distributed throughout foods.) Lecithin naturally present in
egg yolk gives eggs their ability to thicken sauces, custards and
mayonnaise.

There are different types of lecithin: some are extracted from
soyabeans and contain polyunsaturated fats; others come from egg
yolk and have mainly saturated fat. Most of the commercially
available varieties contain around 80 per cent fat, about half of
which is polyunsaturated.

Within the body, lecithin is involved in the transport of fats and is
an essential part of the membrane that surrounds cells. Like
cholesterol, we do not need to eat lecithin since the body is quite
capable of making its own. It is manufactured by the liver from fatty
acids, glycerol (a kind of fat), phosphate and choline (a vitamin-like
substance which is also important for normal brain function). Each
of these ingredients is readily available within the body and there
seems to be no advantage in eating extra lecithin.

When lecithin is taken as a supplement, it is broken down in the
small intestine to its component parts. The extra choline which
comes from eating lecithin may have a role in treating people with
some brain disorders, including senile dementia, but has not been
shown to have benefits for most people.

If you happen to like lecithin granules, remember that they
provide extra fat and are quite high in kilojoules.

TRIGLYCERIDES

After you have eaten a meal, fat is present in the blood in the form
of triglycerides. These should clear after a few hours. High levels
may persist, however, if you have taken in more fat, sugar or alcohol

than your body can use. If you are having a blood test to measure tri-glyceride levels, it should always be performed before breakfast. If the level of triglycerides is high, even after you have had plenty of time for the previous meal to have been cleared from the blood, your risk of heart disease is increased. The debate over whether it is worse to have high levels of cholesterol or triglycerides continues. The consensus is that high levels of either type of fat are undesir-able. To reduce triglyceride levels, sugar, alcohol and too many fats must be avoided.

Fish fats

As we have discussed, there is not much fat in fish and seafoods. However, the small amounts present are rich in omega–3 fatty acids. Research into omega–3s began after it was noticed that the Eskimos seemed to be able to avoid heart disease in spite of a relatively high fat intake from whale and seal fat.

Omega–3 fatty acids have some important virtues. They can:

- reduce the levels of triglycerides in the blood;
- prevent blood clots forming;
- stop certain cells sticking to the walls of the arteries;
- stimulate the growth of smooth-muscle cells in the artery and prevent the thickened clogged artery walls;
- prevent dangerous disturbances to the heart rhythm; and
- help lower blood pressure.

Since a heart attack is usually caused by a blood clot forming in a narrowed artery, fish fats should help prevent heart attacks. Several studies have found that even one to two fish meals a week significantly reduces the risk of heart disease.

Omega–3 fatty acids may also have a role in preventing inflam-mation in the body and providing immunity to certain diseases. Research points to the value of eating fish. It is probably no coincidence that the long-life expectancy of the Japanese is related to the fact that they eat lots of fish and very little saturated fat.

Cold water fish such as salmon and sardines have even more of the omega–3 fatty acids than other fish. The polyunsaturated fats help to prevent the fish from freezing in their very cold environment. Mackerel, tuna and herring also contain omega–3 fatty acids. For those who do not like fish, the omega–3 fatty acids are available in capsules.

HOW TO REDUCE YOUR CHOLESTEROL LEVEL

1   Make sure your weight is in the healthy weight range (see Appendix 1h).

2   Avoid eating too much fat of any kind. Try to keep your total fat for the day down to 20 to 30 per cent of your kilojoules or less (see the table below for specific figures). If you are engaged in a lot of physical activity and therefore need a high kilojoule intake, it will be difficult to reduce fat to below 20 to 25 per cent of kilojoules as the quantities of vegetables, grains and fruits needed will be enormous.

3.   Eat more fish: at least once or twice a week. Fresh or canned fish are suitable but remove oil or brine from canned varieties. Fish oil capsules are a suitable source of omega–3 fatty acids.

4   Eat more fibre. With low–fat high–fibre meals, blood cholesterol levels are likely to be lower. Pectin in fruits and the gummy type of fibre in oats, dried beans and peas are especially valuable.

In general, an average man should aim to keep fat levels below 70 grams a day. For women, an appropriate level would be 50 grams. If you can manage to eat less, by all means do so. Appendix 1a lists more exact levels of fat which are appropriate for those who need to lose weight or have greater levels of physical activity.

Choose your fat

Table 2.1   Fat content of foods

Food	Fat (grams)
Meats	
Large T–bone steak, including fat	48
Lean fillet, small serve	10
Rump steak	33
Mince steak, 150g	24
Pork, forequarter chop, with crackling	54
Pork, loin chop, with no visible fat	4
New-fashioned pork, butterfly steak, no visible fat	5
Lamb loin chops, 2, including fat	45
Roast leg of lamb, no fat, average serve	8
Veal chops, 2	4
Kidneys, average serve	4
Liver, average serve	9
Sausage, 1, grilled	20
Bacon, 2 pieces	30
Meat pie or sausage roll	24
Hamburger	30
Chicken breast, no fat, average serve	3
Turkey, average serve	3
Barbequed chicken, one quarter	15
Chicken, take-away dinner box	51

Table 2.1   Fat content of foods — continued

Food	Fat (grams)
Ham, leg, 60g (amount on a sandwich)	3
Salami, 60g	23
Turkey salami, 60g	3
Seafood	
Fish, with batter, average piece	23
Fish, grilled, average fillet	2
with butter sauce	30
Oysters, 1 dozen, natural	2
Prawns, 4, king size, barbequed	2
Prawns, 4, king size, battered	18
Salmon, canned, 100g	8
Tuna, canned, 100g	4
Hot potato chips, average serve	35
Dairy products	
Milk, 250ml glass	9
Milk, in each cup of tea or coffee	1
Skim, (Shape), 250ml	0
Butter or margarine, on slice of bread	6
Butter or margarine, on hot toast	12
Butter or margarine, 1 tablespoon	16
Cream, average serve	12
Cheese, amount on a sandwich	8
Cottage cheese, half a cup	4
Icecream, rich, 2 scoops	16
regular, average serve	7
Other	
Oil, 1 tablespoon	20
Apple pie, small piece without cream	18
Cheesecake, average serve	45
Chocolate cake, average serve	35
Fruits and vegetables (except avocado)	0
Roast potato, average size	5
Avocado, half	20
Bread, 2 slices	1
Mayonnaise, 1 tablespoon	18
Croissant	14
Egg, 1	6
Savoury biscuits, 4	4
Doughnut	13
Sweet biscuits, 2, plain	5
Potato crisps, small packet	10
Peanuts, 25g	12
Muesli bar	6
Chocolate, 100g	31
Mars bar, 70g size	14

Practical hints for eating less fat

1   Choose seafoods as they contain little fat. Grill, poach or barbecue them to preserve the benefits.

2   With meats, choose turkey, chicken breast, veal, new-fashioned pork, very lean cuts of beef such as fillet or topside, or game (venison, rabbit, hare, pheasant). The leanest cut of lamb is the leg.

3   Choose low-fat processed meats such as turkey ham, or low-fat ham. Try to avoid sausages.

4   Go easy on the spread. Both butter and margarine add heaps of fat. Do you really need either on a freshly cut sandwich?

5   Look for low-fat dairy products such as low-fat fortified milk, skim milk, cottage or ricotta cheeses, and hard cheeses with reduced-fat levels.

6   Keep fatty foods such as chocolates, cream, pastries and cakes for special occasions. Ask yourself if it's worth all that fat before you take a bite. If you restrict yourself to top-quality products, you'll find you automatically eat less.

7   Have a slice or two of wholemeal toast instead of a high-fat croissant.

8   Choose 'no oil' salad dressings and low–fat mayonnaises (or simply use lemon juice and/or fresh herbs on salads).

9   Try a vegetarian meal occasionally. Beans, peas and lentils have stacks of protein, dietary fibre and valuable nutrients, but very little fat.

10   Grill, barbeque, steam, poach, stir fry using concentrated stock, bake on a rack, microwave or wrap food in foil. If you need to fry, use a pan liner.

11   Choose fresh fruit rather than a cheese platter for dessert.

12   Have plenty of fruits, vegetables, breads and cereal products: they have almost no fat and are filling so you won't be looking for fatty foods.

For peak performance

•   Cut fats to an appropriate level for your physical activity (see Appendix 1a for details).

•   Don't allow fats to crowd out the important complex carbohydrates found in breads, cereals, vegetables and legumes.

3

Salt:
Why it causes problems

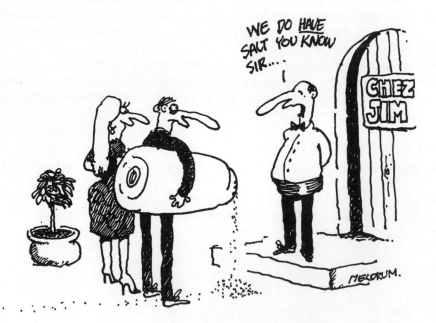

W HY oh why did we ever leave the sea! Almost every land animal has some mechanism for disposing of excess salt, but humans are more like sea creatures and conserve salt in their bodies. Excess levels of the sodium from salt then cause problems with increased blood pressure.

Amphibians can excrete large amounts of salt straight through their skins. Turtles, birds and marine iguanas have a special gland which gets rid of the stuff in nasal secretions. Snakes have a pre–rectal gland to dispose of spare salt, while the camel possesses a wonderful pump which enables it to drink water with twice the salt content of sea water and then to excrete the excess salt. Even the crocodile manages to de–salt itself, not by shedding salty 'crocodile tears', but with special glands on its tongue which can excrete extra salt.

With our inability to cope with a salt overload, humans have failed to adapt to a land environment. Birds' and reptiles' hormones help them offload salt whereas the same hormones in humans tend to hold salt in the body, as if we were sea creatures. Medical researchers sometimes refer to our struggle with salt as 'Neptune's Curse'.

The odium of sodium

Salt is made up of sodium and chlorine, both essential minerals. Sodium has a vital role in controlling the pressure and volume of the blood. It also governs the balance of water inside body cells and in the spaces surrounding the cells. This is particularly important during strenuous physical activity when water is needed inside the cells to allow for energy to be produced. Too much salt pulls the water out of the cells and the energy-producing reactions in the muscle cells cannot function efficiently. Sodium (and potassium, chlorine and magnesium) are termed 'electrolytes' since they are present in the body as electrically charged particles. Their control over the balance of fluids allows dissolved nutrients to enter the cells and waste products to be removed.

The kidneys control the amount of sodium in the body. When we eat too much salt, the kidneys excrete the excess sodium in the urine. After a salty meal, the kidneys need extra water to get rid of the salt and so we feel thirsty. On the other hand, if the level of sodium in the body drops too low, the kidneys stop sodium being lost in the urine and return it to the blood. If you are sweating heavily, and thus losing some extra sodium in your sweat, the kidneys simply reabsorb a little more sodium. Except with kidney failure or after a period of vomiting or diarrhoea, there is no problem in keeping enough sodium in the body. The kidneys are perfectly capable of 27 cutting down on the amount lost in urine. The big problem with sodium is disposing of the excess.

After years of bombarding the body with salty foods and forcing it to get rid of excess salt, the kidneys sometimes malfunction and start to retain too much sodium. This excess sodium then holds extra water in the blood, causing the blood vessels to become waterlogged. Once this occurs, the small blood vessels become overly sensitive to signals which cause them to contract and become tight. The heart then has to work harder to force blood through the narrowed, stiffer blood vessels—and the blood pressure rises.

For most of human history, the problem of disposing of excess sodium and chlorine did not occur; early man's diet contained very little salt. Even today, many tribal and traditional societies consume a diet with no salt apart from the very moderate levels naturally present in foods, and they have wonderfully low blood pressures to show for it. Even though some of these people live in very hot climates, such as in parts of New Guinea, they do not suffer any symptoms of sodium deficiency. The natural sources of sodium are quite sufficient to meet their needs. Their diets also tend to be rich in potassium.

As they grow older, those who have eaten little salt throughout life continue to have the same low blood pressures they enjoyed in their youth. Strokes are unknown. However, if people move from a traditional society into a Western lifestyle, and eat more salt and less potassium, their blood pressure rises and strokes become commonplace.

Most Westerners habitually eat a lot of salt from highly salted processed and fast foods, as well as the salt added to foods during cooking and at the table. An excess of salt has become the norm and the result is high blood pressure with its associated high costs of health care. The drugs to treat the nation's high blood pressure are estimated to cost millions a year. In addition, the medical costs associated with high blood pressure and strokes, as well as the loss of productivity to the community, are enormous. A number of factors is associated with high blood pressure; excessive salt is a major cause.

There are some lucky people who seem to be unaffected by large amounts of salt. You've probably noticed a few healthy-looking octagenarians liberally sprinkling salt over their food with no apparent ill-effects. That does not mean that we can all be so lucky. You may also see people driving like idiots and not having an accident, but you would hardly advise others to follow such an example. Eating excess salt is a health hazard for many people. And if you are one of the fortunate few whose kidneys are not sensitive to added salt, you have no way of knowing that you are a member of such an elite group. Neither will you know how much harm salt is doing to your body—until your blood pressure suddenly rises. It seems crazy to take risks with salt when there is so little to gain and so much to lose by eating an excess.

People with low blood pressure often ask if extra salt might be good for them. Most medical experts do not accept that low blood pressure is a disease unless it is caused by excessive bleeding. Even though high blood pressure will fall when less salt is eaten, a person with normal or low blood pressure will find that eating less salt has no effect. Reducing salt normalises blood pressure.

Salt also has an indirect effect on bones. Strong bones require calcium but the more salt you eat, the greater the loss of calcium in urine. With more calcium being lost, the level of calcium in the blood drops. This in turn increases the secretion of a hormone which withdraws calcium from the bones to restore the blood levels of calcium to normal. If that all sounds a bit complicated, you only need to note that one of the results of eating a lot of salt is a loss of calcium from the bones. Anyone at risk of osteoporosis (a condition of thin, porous bones common in slender women) should therefore avoid eating too much salt.

Salt as a preservative

In spite of its current cheapness, salt was once a highly priced and much-prized commodity. Salt was sometimes traded for gold and a good Greek slave was said to be worth his weight in salt. People who lived in the middle of continents were especially likely to put a high price on salt. Meats, fish, fruits and vegetables could be preserved with salt and such foods could mean the difference between health and semi–starvation. Certainly for the early settlers in Australia, salt pork, salt beef and pickled cabbage were important survival foods. In some parts of the world where refrigeration is not available, salting is still used as a major food processing technique. In such cases, the benefits of salt may well outweigh the disadvantages.

Foods often go 'off' because of bacterial contamination or the formation of mould. Bacteria require a certain amount of moisture. Salt preserves food by altering the moisture, drawing water out so that bacteria and moulds are unable to multiply. The food will then 'keep' longer.

In some foods, such as cheese or pickles, the addition of salt provides the right environment for desirable bacteria to grow and produce the fermentation which result in the final product. In making cheese, for example, salt controls the ripening, provides a firm texture, preserves the cheese and gives it flavour. Too much salt produces a dry, crumbly cheese while too little produces a soft, 29 bland cheese which does not keep for long. Some cheeses, such as blue varieties, have a particularly high salt content so that undesirable bacteria won't survive, but the blue mould, which is relatively salt-resistant, will be able to grow. On the other hand, a cheese such as Swiss, generally has very little salt for a special salt-hating bacteria to produce the characteristic sweet flavour and the 'holes' in the texture.

In some parts of the world, such as in northern Japan, salting of foods is still widely used. Wherever possible, however, salting has been replaced by refrigeration or other methods of food processing since it is now known that those who eat a lot of foods preserved by salting have a high incidence of stomach cancer. Alternative food preservation methods have now made cancer of the stomach rare in Western countries.

Why so much salt?

Salt originally gained its status as a preservative. These days, salt is prized because it can disguise a lack of flavour. With many highly processed foods, much of the taste of the original ingredients is lost during processing. The blandness of the finished product means that ingredients, such as salt and sugar, must be added to provide some semblance of flavour. If you eat fresh foods, carefully prepared to retain their delicious natural taste, you will not need to 'pepper up' your meals with salt. Many highly processed foods, however, need the addition of salt to mask their lack of real flavour.

Salt is also added to many fast foods so that patrons will feel thirsty and buy drinks with their meal. Adding salt also gives a feeling of 'cutting' the greasiness of many fatty fast foods. In fact, the salt simply adds to the problem of fat in such products.

The liking for salt is learned. Babies wrinkle up their noses at their first vegetables, not because they don't like vegetables, but in response to the salt which has usually been added to satisfy an adult's taste buds. It was not until baby food manufacturers carried out taste tests with babies, rather than with babies' mothers, that they realised that infants preferred foods without added salt. Commercial baby foods now have no added salt. However, it is unfortunate that it is only a matter of time before most toddlers are given potato crisps and other salty snack foods and become hooked on salt.

Salt is also used out of habit. Notice how many people sprinkle salt on their meal even before they have tasted it! Once you are accustomed to the taste of salt, it can be difficult to give up. Taste buds which are overloaded with salt take time to adjust to foods without salt. But once the taste buds have adjusted, the natural flavours of foods become more intense. Rather than enhancing the taste, salt simply gives everything a sameness of taste: salty.

Salt and sport

If you lick your arm on a hot day, your sweat may taste salty. Many people remember when soldiers on long route marches, footballers, and those working in a hot environment were given salt tablets. Since sweat contains salt, it was assumed that salt tablets would help to restore losses.

It is now known that a trained athlete loses less salt in sweat than someone who has spasmodic physical activity. This is a further example of the body's ability to conserve sodium. The amount of salt lost in the urine generally is reduced during strenuous physical activity.

With any type of heavy work or exercise, much more water is lost than salt. This means that after heavy sweating the concentration of sodium in the body fluids is increased. It is important to replace fluid losses before taking in extra salt. Salt tablets are particularly undesirable for sportspeople because they further increase the concentration of salt in the body. They also draw too much water into the intestine, causing nausea and vomiting.

Sodium (from salt) controls the amount of water which is inside the cells and in the spaces between cells. When the concentration of sodium in body fluids increases after a heavy sweat, water is drawn out of the cells into the spaces between the cells. Since water is needed inside the cells for the production of energy, taking extra salt before replacing fluid losses can be detrimental to physical performance.

Once the water lost through sweating has been replaced, any salt losses will be easily replenished simply from the normal food supply. Athletes usually eat more food (primarily to obtain more kilojoules) and the extra food eaten automatically supplies more salt. Salt tablets are thus unnecessary for sportspeople. Those given salt tablets have a much higher incidence of high blood pressure later in life than other people of the same age.

Some athletes maintain that they feel like a salty drink after exercise. There is no connection between these 'feelings' and the body's salt requirements. In general, people feel like sweet and/or salty foods for some psychological reason rather than from a physical need.

Salt and cramps

Many people believe that cramps are caused by a lack of salt and that extra salt will cure them. In fact, modern science has found that cramps can occur for many reasons, the most common being a lack of appropriate warm-up for the muscle. A lack of water, or a temporary deficiency of magnesium or potassium or calcium, or the effect of female hormones on these minerals may also be responsible

31

for cramps. But a lack of water is the number one suspect in cases of cramp.

Anyone who is experiencing cramps should make sure that he or she is drinking sufficient water.

Salt, strokes and high blood pressure

Strokes are one of the three most common causes of death, with coronary heart disease and cancer. A stroke (or cerebro–vascular accident) occurs when a blood clot forms in an artery leading to the brain. The harder or stiffer the arteries, and the more fatty deposits present, the more likely the chances of a stroke.

Most people prefer not to think about strokes. They hope that by ignoring such common and nasty events, they will go away, or at least happen only to some other poor soul. Yet it is estimated that strokes cost thousands of millions to Western communities every year.

We know that strokes are caused by high blood pressure (or hypertension). We also know that high blood pressure is more likely when arteries are stiffened or partially clogged by fatty deposits. We also know that being overweight or smoking cigarettes can increase blood pressure. And there is increasing evidence that too much salt raises blood pressure.

Medical researchers have also found that high blood pressure can be reduced very effectively by a strict reduction in the amount of salt eaten. Salt has therefore been incriminated as a major risk factor for high blood pressure.

There are dissenting voices in the case against salt. Several studies have not been able to show that people with high blood pressure consume any more salt than the rest of the population. Others dispute that the average person can cut his or her salt intake far enough to have a significant effect on blood pressure. But most studies point an accusing finger at salt as one of the causes of high blood pressure. Excess weight, too little potassium and calcium, and too much alcohol are also related factors.

How much salt?

The average person takes in 10 to 20 times as much salt as is required. Much of this excess salt comes in processed foods. Some is used in cooking and a further supply is sprinkled on foods at the table. A typical fast food meal of a hamburger and some chips supplies more than half of the day's maximum recommended salt intake, and that's assuming the consumer does not add salt.

heavily processed diet contains more salt than earlier generations have used.

The number of people with high blood pressure could be substantially reduced if we all ate less salt. Chances of high blood pressure are greatest if other members of your family have been affected, or if you are overweight, or have kidney disease, or if you are over 50. On hearing such facts, many people decide that they will worry about their salt intake when they are older. Unfortunately, the damage from salt may have been done many years before that and it makes much better sense to try to cut salt intake to a quantity which is closer to the body's needs for it.

Meat, milk, eggs and some vegetables have a natural content of salt, usually in harmony with the mineral potassium. Other basic foods, such as cheese, require salt during manufacture (it helps to dehydrate the curd and slows the activity of the bacteria which are a vital part of the cheese-making procedure). Unsalted bread can certainly be produced, but the usual addition of salt helps to prevent the wheat protein from being weakened into a sticky mass which will not hold sufficient air. Most breads therefore have salt added and this contributes ample quantities to the daily diet. Simply by eating meat, milk, eggs, vegetables, bread and some cheese, you could easily meet your body's salt requirements. Even without the salt added to bread and cheese, most people would obtain enough salt.

The body's needs for sodium are estimated at 920 to 2300 milligrams per day (2300 milligrams of sodium = 1 millimole). Endurance athletes who are sweating heavily could safely eat twice this amount.

How to eat less salt

You cannot always taste the salt in foods. A bowl of cornflakes, for example, does not taste salty yet it contains more salt than a packet of potato crisps. The crisps taste salty because the salt on the outside of the crisp is immediately apparent to your taste buds. With the cornflakes, the salt is embedded into the product and you are not really aware of an obvious salty flavour.

Knowing the salt content of foods can be confusing too. Vegemite, for example, contains about 8 grams of salt per 100 grams of the product or 3200 milligrams of sodium in 100 grams: a horrific-sounding amount. However, an average spread of Vegemite on a slice of bread contains just 110 milligrams of sodium: less than the quantity of salt in the slice of bread.

Some people find it easiest to give up salt by going cold turkey: they simply stop salting food and avoid items with a high salt content. If you can manage such a drastic change, that's fine. But 33 most people who try this method decide that saltless food is too bland and revert to using salt. Most people's taste buds take time to adjust and studies in the United States have found that there is usually a greater chance of success if salt is given up gradually.

A recent study provided evidence that after giving up salt, subjects no longer liked salty foods. Five months after giving up salt, participants were given the same foods which they had previously enjoyed. They now rated these foods as unpleasantly salty. However, the same researchers found that after three weeks on the low-salt foods, most people found salt exceptionally pleasant. They concluded that there is a critical period, possibly two months, before the liking for salt changes to dislike.

Giving up the salt shaker may not be the best way to start on the low-salt way of life. The salt which you add last really hits your taste buds. Its absence can be painfully obvious. On the other hand, the salt used in cooking can be gradually reduced without being noticed. You might think that as the salt in the cooking is reduced there will be a corresponding increase in the salt sprinkled on at the table. The great majority of people pick up a salt shaker and sprinkle salt onto their food for a set length of time. In most cases, they do not taste the food first, and they rarely add more salt once they begin eating the meal. An Australian study found that the amount of salt added to foods was in direct proportion to the size of the holes in the salt shakers! Unbeknown to them, people were observed eating and their salt consumption was measured. When the holes in the salt shakers were partly 'gummed up', they simply ate less salt. If you completely block off the holes, it will be noticed! But as long as some salt comes out, most people will sprinkle for a set length of time rather than for a certain level of saltiness. Salting food is thus a habit which has been learned. It can also be 'unlearned'.

Start by using about three-quarters of the amount of salt you usually use in cooking. After about a week, cut down to half then follow this with further reductions. It may take weeks, but your palate will adjust to foods with less salt. Some people don't want to start eating less salt because they do not like the thought of eating one or two particular foods without salt. It there are foods, such as eggs or tomatoes, on which you particularly like salt, keep salting these foods in your usual fashion for the time being. As you reduce the amount of salt you're using on other foods, you'll find you prefer less, even on items you previously loved with added salt. By cutting back on the salt added to the majority of your foods, you'll be doing your body a great favour.

The more taste a food has, the less salt needs to be added. The idea that salt 'brings out' the flavour in foods is disputed by many who have given up adding salt. Once their taste buds have recovered

34

from their previous salt assault, these people report that the natural flavours of foods are now clearer since they are not uniformly distorted by salt.

While you are using less salt, you could also take a look at your cooking methods.

The role of potassium

The sodium from salt should ideally be balanced with potassium from foods. In natural foods, potassium is present at far higher levels than sodium. Many processed foods, however, have lost some of their natural potassium and gained large quantities of sodium from salt. This distorts the natural balance of these two minerals. For example, a fresh tomato has more than 50 times as much potassium as sodium; canned tomatoes have only one tenth of this quantity while the more highly processed tomato sauce has almost twice as much sodium as potassium.

Fruits and vegetables are excellent sources of potassium (dried fruits are exceptionally rich). Fresh meats and poultry have more potassium than sodium but this is reversed with processed varieties. Grains are also rich in potassium and low in sodium; most prepared breakfast cereals and bread have more sodium. Potassium-rich foods can help balance some of the salt that we cannot always avoid. For example, a salad sandwich and some fresh fruit will contain plenty of potassium to balance the salt which has been used in making the bread.

Salt substitutes

A variety of salt substitutes are available to ease the move into the low-salt lifestyle. Most contain potassium chloride in place of some or all of the regular sodium chloride. To some people, potassium chloride leaves an unpleasant bitter flavour; others find it perfectly acceptable.

Salt substitutes can be useful but most people find it simpler to gradually use less salt. The bonus in adjusting the taste buds to less salt is that the true flavours of foods become more enjoyable.

Salt substitutes can be dangerous for anyone with kidney problems. It is also important to note that some products still contain 50 per cent salt.

Sea salt is sometimes sold as an alternative to regular salt. It is still sodium chloride and has absolutely no advantages. Don't waste your money on it and don't expect any benefits.

Vegetable salts are also promoted as a healthy alternative to regular salt. These products are still based on salt but have various vegetable extracts added to provide extra flavour. They too offer little health advantage over ordinary salt and won't do a thing for your blood pressure.

Practical hints for cutting down on salt

1. Gradually use less salt in cooking until you are able to enjoy the natural flavours of foods without added salt. Follow this with a gradual reduction in the salt used at the table.
2. Always taste food *before* using salt.
3. Use very little water when cooking vegetables. The more water you use, the more the flavour will dissolve into the water.
4. Use a microwave, if available. Microwaved vegetables have much more flavour because they can be cooked with little or no water. They taste great without salt.
5. Use herbs (fresh or dried) to add an extra dimension of taste to foods (see the herb chart, Appendix 1f to mix and match flavours).
6. Use spices when cooking casseroles, meat, chicken and fish dishes.
7. Snack on fresh fruits, crisp raw vegetables, fruit loaf, unsalted crackers, unsalted nuts or pepitas (varieties of roasted pumpkin seeds), or hot freshly popped corn with mixed dried salad herbs. Avoid packets of salty snacks.
8. Choose fresh rather than processed meats. Sausages, salamis and cured meats have lots of added salt.
9. Try brown rice rather than white. The nuttier flavour makes salt less necessary.
10. Look for unsalted canned foods (almost every canned product is now available in an unsalted version). Start off with unsalted tomato products used in recipes which have plenty of flavour from herbs and/or spices.
11. Try unsalted butter or margarine (it's surprising how fast the regular varieties begin to taste unpleasantly salty). Look for peanut butter without salt, unsalted crackers, no added salt sauces and soups.
12. Use an untoasted muesli (or make your own, see recipe in Appendix 1e or try puffed wheat or one of the breakfast cereals marked 'no added salt'.
13. Porridge and soups are two foods which really taste different without salt. Try adding some raisins or sultanas or a few unsalted pepitas to porridge. With soups, use a good strong home-made chicken stock and plenty of herbs to add flavour.
14. Use a dash of lemon juice to add flavour to meat, fish, vegetables and pasta recipes. A little finely grated orange or lemon rind also perks up the flavour of many foods.

36

For peak performance

- Avoid eating a lot of salt (see practical hints, this chapter).
- Endurance athletes can take in more salt than other people but it is still desirable to avoid excess quantities.
- Eat plenty of potassium-rich foods such as fresh and dried fruits, vegetables and grains.

4

Sugar:
How much is too much?

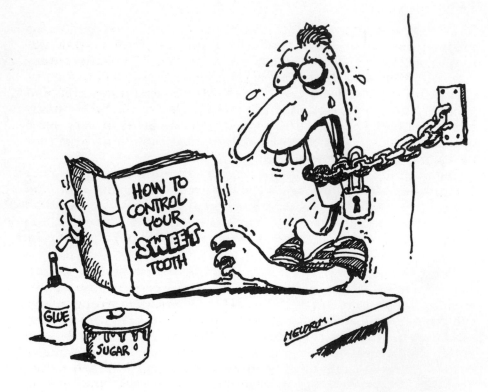

AS the sugar industry loves to remind us, sugar cane grows quite naturally. Millions of dollars are spent in a grand advertising effort to convince us that the white crystals which are added to most foods are 'a natural part of life'. Antagonists of sugar, on the other hand, refer to sugar as being 'pure, white and deadly'.

The sugar cane is certainly natural, but the processing which removes every vestige of protein, dietary fibre, minerals and vitamins is not. Sugar may taste nice but there is no nutritional reason why anyone should eat it. By the same token, if you like sugar (and most people instinctively do), a little will do no harm. The 'deadly' accusations are difficult to uphold. However, sugar can create problems when it is eaten in excessive amounts, and consumption in countries like Australia is alarmingly high.

The history of sugar

Sugar was not always 'a natural part of life'. The technique for pressing out the juice and boiling it down into dark crystals was developed in India around 500 BC. It was not until the sixth century AD, however, that both the sugar cane and the technique for extracting its juice were taken to the Tigris–Euphrates area and then to North Africa, Spain and Syria. By the fourteenth century, sugar was being shipped to England, but was used in very small quantities as a flavouring and as a drug. It also found widespread use in making various medicines more palatable.

Sugar gradually moved from being a medicine to a luxury product, usually in the form of a syrup around nuts and seeds, and later in cakes. By the eighteenth century, sugar consumption had increased to two kilograms a year. The wealthier you were, the more sugar you were likely to eat. Honey was also popular but, like sugar, it was expensive.

The European craving for sugar became so strong that, during the eighteenth century, millions of Africans were forced into slavery to cultivate sugar cane in the West Indies. There was a strong reason for the new popularity of sugar in Europe. The 17th century had seen three new products introduced to Europe. Each of these—tea, coffee and chocolate—were preferred with sugar. Interestingly, none of these beverages had been served sweetened in their native countries. In Europe, they were preferred with sugar and milk or cream added.

With the growing popularity of sugar, the sugar industry became the major force behind the slave trade with more than two-thirds of the 20 million African slaves working on sugar plantations. Rum, made cheaply from the by-products of sugar cane, also entered the

39

grim picture of slavery and corruption. This was the first mass-produced spirit made from the residues of sugar refining, mixed with molasses, fermented and distilled. The enormous fortunes made by the owners of sugar plantations and rum distilleries then began to finance the Industrial Revolution. It is probably fair to say that no food has rivalled sugar for its influence on human affairs.

The first real barb in the war against the dominance of sugar cane came in the eighteenth century when a Prussian chemist developed a method of isolating sugar crystals from sugar beet. During the 1800s, sugar-beet factories sprang up all over Europe and the sugar beet now accounts for 40 per cent of the sugar produced in the world.

In more recent times in the United States, corn has also challenged sugar because it can be converted to a sweet substance known as high-fructose corn syrup. This accounts for nearly half of the total sugar supply in the United States.

The latest challenge to the sugar industry is coming from other sweeteners. Unlike the early artificial sweeteners, saccharin and cyclamates, the more recently developed sweeteners taste so much like sugar that few people can pick the difference.

What is wrong with sugar?

Sugar's best documented vice is its effect on teeth. Its total effects on the human body are much more difficult to assess. In evolutionary terms, sugar is a very recent addition to the human diet. If we imagine the whole of human existence being condensed to a 24–hour time span, the period of high sugar consumption represents only a few seconds. It may be that insufficient time has elapsed for the human body to become accustomed to being bombarded with so much sugar.

Most health authorities now believe that it is excess quantities of sugar which cause health problems. The major controversies centre on a definition of excess. For most of the last 40 years or so, Westerners have managed to down an average of 40–50 kilograms of sugar a year. Over the last few years, however, sugar consumption has been falling slightly as health authorities have convinced consumers that current consumption is too high. The sweet addiction was providing too many kilojoules for a community with little physical activity. However, as a result of vigorous advertising to combat the effects of the health message, it appears that domestic sugar consumption is increasing.

It is difficult to point the finger directly at sugar. Small to moderate quantities seem to do no harm. Even with the kilogram or so that is currently being eaten each week, it is hard to single out any specific effects of sugar, apart from its damaging effect on teeth. Much of the sugar we eat comes in foods which are also high in fat, and lacking important nutrients and dietary fibre. Which is the real culprit? The sugar? The fat? The lack of fibre?

Sugar and dental decay

There is no controversy about sugar and dental decay. Even the sugar industry admits that sugar plays a major role in dental caries although, having acknowledged this, they tend to brush the fact aside, failing to see the enormous health implications of this damage. Dentists are more outspoken and claim that dental decay is the major public health problem. It may not be life-threatening but holes in the teeth are entirely preventable.

Sugar and obesity

Other harmful effects of sugar are difficult to prove. Some maintain that sugar itself does not cause obesity. However, in a country with more than a third of men and women being regarded as overweight (more men than women), the large number of kilojoules being provided by a nutritionally useless food such as sugar must provoke criticism. Excess sugar, like an excess of most foods, contributes to the national girth.

The average sugar intake contributes 14 000–15 000 kilojoules (approximately 3500 Calories) a week and, as many people have discovered, when you stop eating sugar and sweet foods, you lose weight. Some of this comes from the reduction of the fat which accompanies the sugar.

Some people eat less than the average weekly consumption of sugar, which means that others munch their way through even more than that. Nutritionists are concerned at all these 'empty' calories (that is, calories which are unaccompanied by any essential nutrients). That is why dietary recommendations state 'avoid eating too much sugar'.

The major problem lies in establishing a safe sugar intake. Some people are more sugar-sensitive than others. For these people, one study found that limiting sugar to 5 per cent of their total kilojoules was beneficial. For the average woman, this would be equivalent to eating about 25 grams of sugar a day; for men 30 to 35 grams a day. Body frame size and amount of body fat, consideration of other foods eaten and the level of physical activity are also important in determining an appropriate level of sugar. There is no doubt, however, that the balance of our diet would improve if we reduced our current high average intake.

41

Sugar and fat frequently go together. Cakes, pastries, biscuits, desserts, chocolates and some types of confectionery contain both. Most would not be eaten if their sugar was removed.

Some studies have shown that eating sugar at levels typically consumed in Western countries will cause the body to produce more insulin. This alters the levels of fats in the blood. For athletes, it has been shown that sugar triggers a response in the liver which prevents glucose from getting to the muscles where it is needed.

The sweet addiction also means that sugary items of low nutritional value are often chosen in preference to more nutritious foods, particularly by children. An Australian study showed that about 30 per cent of Australian children eat no fruit and a further 30 per cent eat only one piece a day. Bread consumption is low and more than two-thirds of children fail to drink sufficient milk to provide calcium for their growing bones. Yet for the average child sugar now contributes 25 per cent of the kilojoules. Children are choosing sugary foods, and neglecting the nutritious foods that their growing bodies need. Some adults are in a similar position : rejecting foods such as fruit in favour of confectionery items.

Sugar slips down so effortlessly that it is not filling. With every vestige of its dietary fibre stripped off, sugar can be added to foods, increasing their energy density without significantly altering their satiety value. This is ideal for a food industry which wants people to consume more. After all, if you eat foods which are filling, you stop eating sooner. If foods don't really fill you up, you can shovel far more into your body—and make more profits for their manufacturers.

Too many people ignore the more filling foods and go for the easy eating option. The price is an unbalanced diet, and an expanding waistline.

Sugar has been accused of causing hyperactivity. Most parents who experience the horrors of children's behaviour after a party are convinced that sugar and/or the colourings in foods are to blame. However, properly controlled studies have failed to confirm this popular belief. In some criminal institutions in the United States, social workers have claimed that improvements in the diet, which have included replacing sugary foods with more nutritious alternatives, have improved behaviour. Others claim that it is the extra care and attention being given to the people in these institutions which is responsible.

Researchers have also been unable to prove that sugar causes diabetes, although there is plenty of evidence that anyone who has diabetes will find it easier to control their condition if sugar is cut to a minimum. The role of sugar in causing diabetes may be confined to its contribution to excess weight. Once excess weight is lost, type

II diabetes often disappears. The role of sugar in causing heart disease is probably also related to unnecessary kilojoules.

In summary, the only real charges which can be levelled at sugar are that it:

- causes dental decay, unless teeth are thoroughly cleaned after each time that sugar is consumed;
- makes fats more palatable;
- tends to displace other more nutritious foods from the diet; and
- may create a special sensitivity in some people and may cause an increase in levels of some blood fats if sugar intake is too high.

Sugar: where is it hidden?

Until fairly recently, people tended to have some idea of how much sugar they were eating. Most foods were prepared in the home kitchen and the housewife was aware of how often the sugar canister was empty. These days more than 80 per cent of all sugar consumed comes from processed foods.

Sugar lurks in some of the most unlikely places. You expect to find sugar in jams and jellies, cakes and pastries and confectionery, but would you have guessed its presence in peanut butter, some yeast extracts, mayonnaise and salad dressings, canned and packet soups, tomato sauce, baked beans and canned vegetables, many savoury biscuits, stock cubes and hamburger buns? Sugar makes up a major part of some breakfast cereals while every can of soft drink (apart from the low-kilojoule varieties) contains between seven and twelve teaspoons of sugar. And then there is the sugar added to frozen desserts, iceblocks, yoghurt, fruit juices and fruit juice drinks. Sugar also retains its role in sweetening medicines and pills and the earnest vitamin pill-popper can take in quite a bit of sugar.

The largest single source of sugar in the diet of most Western countries is non–alcoholic beverages. Confectionery, preserved foods, purchased cakes, biscuits, breakfast cereals, jams and alcoholic beverages each account for a significant percentage of our total consumption.

Different types of sugars

Sugar from sugar cane is more properly termed sucrose. Other sugars exit as:

Glucose (also known as dextrose): found in small quantities in fruits, vegetables and honey. All other sugars and complex carbohydrates are eventually broken down to glucose.

43

Lactose: found naturally in milk. Breast milk has a higher content than cow's milk.

Fructose: found in fruits and honey. It is the sweetest of the carbohydrate sugars.

Maltose: found in sprouting grains and malt.

Sucrose itself can exist as molasses, treacle, raw sugar, golden syrup, brown sugar, regular white sugar, caster sugar or the finely ground icing sugar. There is also honey which is a mixture of glucose, fructose and water with small quantities of sucrose, other sugars, minerals and acids.

In terms of nutritional value, all sugars contribute 16 kilojoules per gram (or 4 Calories per gram): less than half the number provided by fats. Most forms of sugar in common use have negligible quantities of nutrients present.

Fructose (fruit sugar) is sometimes promoted as a healthier alternative sugar. In cold drinks, fructose certainly tastes sweeter than sucrose and therefore less is required. It has also been found that fructose is slightly less harmful to teeth than regular sucrose. However, any advantages that fructose has do not justify the high price which some people pay for this product. Fructose is best eaten in its truly natural form : fruit.

Lactose is used to sweeten babies' milk mixtures. As it tastes less sweet than regular sugar, it is less likely to promote a sweet tooth in the infant. Breast milk contains much more lactose than cow's or goat's milk.

The problem with food labels

One of the major problems with sugar is that food labels do not require manufacturers to list the percentage of added sugar. If we knew that a product contained 10 or 45 per cent sugar, we could at least make an informed choice. We may well ask why food manufacturers are so reluctant to tell us the amount of sugar added to a product. The usual response is that consumers would be confused by such information! Food manufacturers also maintain that they add so much sugar to products because 'consumers want it'. If consumers are so keen to have lots of sugar, why not splash across the package 'our product has X per cent sugar'. In reality, most food manufacturers would rather not let consumers know how much sugar some products contain because they fear a consumer backlash.

On the label of any food package, ingredients must be listed in their order of predominance (by weight). For some products, this means that sugar should be listed as the first or second ingredient.

44

Some food manufacturers will therefore use several different kinds of sugars so that each one will be present in a smaller proportion and will not be seen as the major ingredient in the product. For example, if a so-called apricot 'health' bar consists of 60 per cent sugar and 40 per cent apricots, it would have to list sugar as its major ingredient. But if the manufacturer puts in 20 per cent of each of three different sugars, the apricots can be listed as the major ingredient. Take a look at the ingredient list on some packets of breakfast cereals and count up how many sugars are present. If there are a number of sugars listed (look for words ending in 'ose' as well as sugar, honey or raw sugar), it's a reasonable assumption that the total sugar content in the product is high.

Other sweeteners

Sucrose, or regular sugar, tastes sweet. But there are many other substances which leave it for dead in this regard. Some other sweeteners are discussed below.

Honey, a sweetener prized and loved for centuries consists of a mixture of fructose and glucose with a small amount of sucrose. It is often regarded as a 'health food' but contains such tiny quantities of minerals and vitamins that they are insignificant in the total diet. The claims that honey is 'natural' ignore the fact that honey is a natural sugar for bees rather than for humans. The nutrients present are quite significant for something the size of the bee. Some wild Australian bush honeys, however, have been found to contain quite significant amounts of nutrients and may well have been an important source of certain amino acids (components of protein) in the diet of Aborigines.

Molasses, an early by-product in the refining of sugar contains reasonable quantities of some minerals, especially calcium, iron and chromium. Two tablespoons of molasses would supply approximately 25 per cent of a woman's daily iron and calcium requirements. It is also a source of potassium and still retains some of the original B-complex vitamins of the sugar cane. Contrary to some health food devotees, the minerals in molasses can be easily obtained from other more palatable foods which are less harmful to the teeth.

As sugar becomes more refined, the nutrients present decrease. Treacle has much smaller quantities of nutrients. Golden syrup contains only a fraction of the iron of molasses and much less calcium. Brown sugar has lost still more of the nutrients and contains virtually no vitamins. And the modern-day raw sugar has little nutritional advantage over white sugar. The only nutrient left in raw sugar may be traces of chromium, a mineral which is involved

45

in the action of insulin within the body. In general, though, there is little advantage in eating raw sugar.

Corn sweeteners are produced by converting the complex carbohydrate in the corn into glucose and then into the sweeter fructose sugar. These sweeteners are cheap to produce and are widely used in the United States but are not used to any great extent in other Western countries.

Sugar alcohols (including sorbitol, mannitol, xylitol) are less sweet than regular sugar but are sometimes used as sugar substitutes in foods such as syrups, low-kilojoule jellies, jams and jubes. They are used to give 'body' to these products. Since sugar alcohols do not need insulin to be used by the body, they were once proposed as suitable products for diabetics. However, since the sugar alcohols still contribute kilojoules, they are of limited benefit to diabetics. They are kinder to teeth than sugar but in large quantites they cause diarrhoea.

Certain teas and shrubs contain sweet substances which are used by small groups of people in primitive societies. Some are used in food products in Japan.

An extract of licorice has a taste which is about 50 times as sweet as sugar. It is used in some types of confectionery, in liqueurs, chocolate and in vanilla flavourings.

Various fruits, including the Lo Han Fruit in Southern China, contain sweet substances which are up to 400 times as sweet as sugar.

Protein sweeteners also exist in nature. The serendipity berry which grows in tropical West Africa contains a protein which is about 2500 times sweeter than sugar. The miracle fruit, another native African fruit, contains a substance at the base of its seeds which is several thousand times as sweet as sugar. This substance is sold in the United States and in Japan. It has been used by native populations for hundreds of years to make sour-tasting foods, such as lemons, taste delightfully sweet.

Artificial sweeteners began with the discovery of saccharin in 1879. This substance leaves a slightly bitter aftertaste but has been used by diabetics for much of this century. Cyclamate sweeteners have more recently been added to the diabetic's sweetening list. Both these substances have been subject to bans in the United States because they have been found to cause cancer of the bladder in certain strains of rats. The concentration needed to produce the cancer was equivalent to a human drinking some 800 cups of artificially sweetened liquid a day! There really is no evidence that the small quantities usually consumed have any harmful effects. It is likely that almost any substance fed in such concentrations will be harmful. Sugar would certainly overstrain the ability of the pancreas to cope if given in such a load.

Newer sweeteners, such as aspartame (sold as Equal or as the food ingredient NutraSweet), have been thoroughly tested before being permitted as a food ingredient. Aspartame is made from two amino acids (components of protein), neither of which taste sweet when apart, but together are 200 times as sweet as sugar. Each of the amino acids, phenylalanine and aspartic acid, are found naturally in almost every food we eat. Unlike saccharin and cyclamates, which taste sweet in the mouth and are then excreted by the body, the amino acids in aspartame are digested like any other amino acid. This sweetener is thus more 'natural' in its action than previous sweeteners. The taste of aspartame is so much like sugar that most people are unable to distinguish between the two. Because it is less bulky than sugar, and is easier to transport and store, it is increasingly being used in products such as soft drinks. In some countries, such as Canada, it is the only artificial sweetener permitted.

In spite of over 100 tests regarding its safety, aspartame has its critics. Naturally, the sugar industry is upset with its success. Others have pointed out the dangers of aspartame to people with the rare genetic disorder called phenylketonuria (PKU). These people must begin life on a completely artificial diet and, throughout life, have to strictly limit any source of protein such as meat, eggs, cheese, fish or milk since a build–up of phenylalanine causes brain dysfunction and retardation. For this group of people, a special warning is printed on products containing aspartame. Some people misinterpret research relating to this group of people and assume that phenylalanine is harmful for the whole population. It is not.

Acesulfame K is another protein sweetener which is likely to be used in foods in the future.

The sweetest known compound is 33 000 times as sweet as sugar. One grain too much, and you'd ruin the cake!

Sugar and sports performance

Many people believe that glucose or sugar taken just before a sporting event will provide instant energy. It won't. There is no such thing as quick energy. The energy in the muscles is present in the form of glycogen and is a result of what was eaten many hours beforehand. What you ate yesterday is much more important than any quick snack before an event. Taking sugar or glucose just before an event can actually be a hindrance to optimal performance. When sugar is eaten, it is goes into the stomach where it stays for varying lengths of time depending on what else has been eaten. Tension will delay the emptying of the stomach. While in the stomach, the sugar will draw water from the tissues into the stomach to dilute the sugar.

This is undesirable since plenty of water is needed in the body's tissues rather than in the stomach.

Some time after sugar is eaten, it leaves the stomach and passes into the small intestine. Here it is broken down to glucose and fructose which are then absorbed into the blood. Once glucose enters the blood, the pancreas produces insulin which helps the sugar pass from the blood into the muscles. (In untreated diabetics with insufficient insulin, the glucose cannot get into the muscles and the level of glucose in the blood rises until the excess 'spills over' into the urine.) If you take glucose or sugar just before exercise, the insulin level in the blood will rise and remain high for an hour or two. The purpose of the extra insulin is to increase the rate at which glucose is removed from the blood. If you begin to exercise during this period, the insulin can remove too much of the sugar from the blood, causing a lower than usual blood sugar level. When this occurs, reaction times can falter, judgement can be temporarily impaired and a feeling of fatigue sets in.

Too much insulin can also interfere with the body's ability to mobilise fatty acids as a source of energy. For anyone involved in a long run or other endurance exercise, a lowered ability to use fat for energy means that muscle glycogen stores will be used up faster, leading to exhaustion.

Once you begin to exercise, the amount of insulin produced is controlled by the exercise itself. For endurance athletes, therefore, sugar can be taken once exercise begins. But it is unwise to take sugar, glucose or glucose drinks just prior to exercise. It will not give you instant energy.

Sugar is a carbohydrate and some athletes therefore think that eating more sugar is a good idea. However, sugar, unlike the carbohydrates found in breads, cereals, grains, legumes, fruits and vegetables, does not contain the minerals and vitamins needed for its carbohydrate to be used by the body.

How much sugar?

It is unrealistic to expect people to do without sugar. Nor does it appear to be necessary. However, there are some general guidelines.

Energy needs are falling as people become more sedentary and do less physical work. However, the body's needs for iron or calcium or protein or dietary fibre or most other nutrients is not changing to any extent. It is therefore logical that we should retain those foods which supply the essential nutrients with their kilojoules and decrease those which provide kilojoules but nothing else. Sugar is thus an example of a food which we should be decreasing.

48

Most nutritionists would be happy if sugar consumption could be halved with an increase in breads, cereals, fruits and vegetables to provide carbohydrate plus other nutrients and dietary fibre. You don't really need to eat any sugar at all. Since the social side of eating is difficult with no sugar, a more rational approach is to keep sugar to a minimum.

An appropriate daily level of kilojoules to be provided from sugar for an adult is 5–10 per cent. For the average man, this equates to a daily sugar intake of 30 to 60 grams. An appropriate level for the average woman would be 25 to 45 grams. If you choose to eat less sugar than this, or even none at all, your diet will not suffer. Without sugar, more of your day's food can come in a nutritionally useful form.

Those who are overweight should cut sugar to a minimum. Anyone who is physically active can generally manage to take in a little more sugar than those who lead sedentary lives. However, even those who are very active should ensure that sugar does not displace more nutritious foods.

Sugar content of foods

Many foods contain only small quantities of sugar. To allow for these inevitable contributions, and to reduce the burden of including them all, assume that about 5 to 10 grams will be contributed by items such as soups, sauces, canned vegetables, salad dressings and various recipe ingredients.

Table 4.1 Sugar content of foods

Food	Sugar content (grams)
Level teaspoon	4
Typical sugar spoon (as added to tea, coffee)	8
Soft drinks, 1 can	40
Flavoured mineral water, 1 can	30
Flavoured milk, 300mL	12
Fruit juice, 250mL	10
Thick shake, average	25
Chocolate flavouring, 1 tablespoon	13
Chocolate powder flavouring, 1 teaspoon	5
Icecream, average serve	14
Iceblocks, average	16
Flavoured yoghurt, 200g	18
Cake, iced, 1 slice	30
Apple pie, 1 small	11
Canned fruit, average serve	16
Jelly, average serve	18
Custard, average serve	10

Table 4.1   Sugar content of foods — continued

Food	Sugar content (grams)
Biscuits, chocolate, 2	9
cream-filled, 2	10
plain, sweet, 2	6
Chocolate biscuit-type bar	18
Health bars, average	11
Toffee, 30g	20
Lollies, each	5
Chocolate, 4 squares	16
Jam or honey (amount on a slice of toast)	10
Breakfast cereals	
Allbran, 50g	8
Branflakes, 50g	7
Cornflakes, 30g (small serve)	3
Coco pops, 30g (small serve)	12
FibrePlus	5
Just Right, 30g	9
Life Be In It, 30g	1
Muesli, toasted, small serve	12
plain, small serve	10
Nutrigrain, 50g	10
Puffed wheat, 30g	1
Readyweets, 50g	1
Rice Bubbles, 30g	3
Special K, 30g	5
Sustain, 50g	7
Weetabix or Vita Brits, 2	1

Practical hints for eating less sugar

1   Choose porridge or a low-sugar/high-fibre breakfast cereal.
2   If you like your cereal sweetened, add a sliced banana or some sultanas or use an artificial sweetener.
3   Gradually reduce the sugar you add to tea and coffee (or switch to an artificial sweetener, preferably one of the new varieties).
4   If you need to eat morning tea, have some fresh or dried fruits or some low-fat cheese with wholegrain wheat or rye crispbread or some bread or muffins.
5   Drink water in place of sweetened drinks.
6   Choose low-kilojoule soft drinks or plain mineral water when you want a fizzy drink.
7   Have fresh fruit for dessert, at least most of the time.

For peak performance

• Sweet foods should not be consumed within an hour prior to an athletic or sports event.

- Do not let sweet foods displace the less refined carbohydrates such as breads, cereals (preferably wholegrain), fruits, potatoes, beans and other vegetables.
- In general try to keep sugar to 5 to 10 per cent of your day's kilojoules.
- Anyone who is overweight should use minimal quantities of both fats and sugar.
- Sweet foods and drinks should be restricted to those times when teeth can be brushed. For this reason, sweet foods are not recommended for sale in school tuckshops or between sporting events.

5

Complex carbohydrates:
The joy of eating more

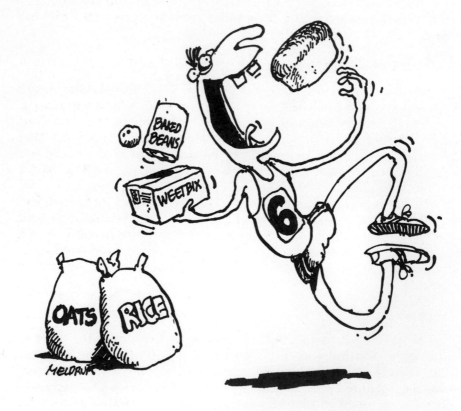

FOR years, bread and potatoes have been shunned for being 'fattening'. Believing they were doing the right thing, many people have been decreasing their consumption of these nutritious foods. Somewhat ironically, as people have been eating less of what they think are waist-expanding foods, the population has been growing steadily fatter.

Bread and potatoes contain complex carbohydrates, so named because they are complex molecules made up of thousands of glucose units. These carbohydrates occur in all cereal and grain foods, in products such as pasta, in vegetables and in legumes (dried peas, beans and lentils). A few fruits, such as bananas, also contain some complex carbohydrate.

Westerners have traditionally eaten most of their complex carbohydrates in the form of bread and potatoes. Most grains, with the exception of rice, have never featured in our culinary repertoire and few people have eaten legumes, mainly because they do not know how to cook them. So the demise of bread and potatoes has meant that the total amount of complex carbohydrate in the diet has fallen.

How much are we eating?

In Australia the recent National Dietary Survey of Adults found that men average just four slices of bread a day while women eat only 2.5 slices. Potato consumption in both groups was very low. Other studies of Australian eating habits have reported that complex carbohydrate makes up just 17 per cent of adults' diets, and only 15 per cent of adolescents' daily food intake. In the UK 20 per cent of energy intake comes from complex carbohydrate.

Current recommendations are that complex carbohydrates should be the major component of the daily diet, making up at least 45 to 50 per cent of the day's kilojoules. Yet until we in the Western world dispel the notion that complex carbohydrates are fattening, it will be difficult to increase the consumption of these important foods.

Starches?

One of the basic problems of complex carbohydrates is their frequent association with fat. Until recently, foods such as breads, potatoes and cereal products were classified as 'starches'. Starchy foods also included pies, sausage rolls, doughnuts and pastries: foods which have more kilojoules coming from fat than from carbohydrate.

In an attempt to dissociate the valuable carbohydrate foods from these fatty foods, the more technically correct term 'complex   53 carbohydrate' is preferable for foods such as breads of all types, all grains, many breakfast cereals and pasta.

Old habits die hard however, and most people still believe that they should restrict their intake of complex carbohydrates for fear of growing fat. Many people who will not eat a potato will munch their way through a packet of potato crisps, with seven times as many kilojoules as potato!

There are encouraging signs that people are beginning to change their attitude towards complex carbohydrates. The Pritikin diet, which allows unlimited quantities of complex carbohydrate (and produces rather thin devotees), has helped. Many sportspeople have also adopted a diet high in complex carbohydrate and discovered improved performance and a greater ability to control their body weight. Many other people have found that a diet with more complex carbohydrate and less fat helps them to achieve greatly reduced levels of cholesterol in their blood. These experiences of the benefits of complex carbohydrates are beginning to filter through to the rest of the population.

A stigma against complex carbohydrates has also existed because many of these foods are reasonably cheap. The most expensive foods are not necessarily the most nutritious. Most of the world's population lives cheaply and healthily on inexpensive sources of complex carbohydrate. The Western world's rejection of such foods in favour of more expensive animal products is to its detriment.

Complex carbohydrates and exercise

Anyone who is trying to exercise, and eats a typical Western diet, will find exercise difficult. Those who eat insufficient quantities of complex carbohydrate foods, such as bread and potatoes, are depriving their bodies of the full potential for physical activity. Many people begin an exercise programme and then give up, claiming that exercise makes them tired. It is usually not the exercise which is to blame, but the unbalanced diet that they are following which fails to provide the appropriate fuel for exercise. With a high fat diet, similar to that eaten in most Western countries, capacity for physical activity is low.

Slimmers who try to exercise are especially likely to find physical activity tiring since most weight reduction diets are even more deficient in complex carbohydrate than the regular fare. A few of the recent and better-balanced slimming diets have realised the value of including sufficient complex carbohydrate so that exercise is possible.

Plenty of carbohydrate allows muscles to be used for a much longer time before they reach exhaustion.

Over a 24-hour period, the type of carbohydrate eaten does not make a great deal of difference in enabling muscles to produce energy. In the longer term, however, complex carbohydrates produce the best fuel for the muscles.

When carbohydrates are eaten and digested, the glucose becomes available for fuel for the muscles. Why not just eat glucose? To answer that, we must look at the process of digestion and also consider the balance of other nutrients provided by the foods which are sources of complex carbohydrates.

Digestion and carbohydrates

The digestion of complex carbohydrates begins in the mouth. Thorough chewing allows an enzyme in saliva to begin to split carbohydrates. Once swallowed, food passes into the stomach where it is held for some time before being ejected in small spurts into the small intestine.

While in the stomach, the food is mixed with hydrochloric acid, and some proteins begin to be broken down. The acidity of the stomach is quite normal and is essential for the digestion of food. Some popular (but unqualified) nutrition writers have recently suggested that mixing foods such as fruits and proteins causes food to 'ferment' in the acid of the stomach. As anyone who has studied basic biochemistry could explain, such notions are ridiculous. The human intestine is ideally built to cope with mixtures of protein, fat and carbohydrate.

Most foods consist of mixtures of various nutrients. We may refer to bread or potatoes as 'complex carbohydrate' foods, but they also contain some protein and very small quantities of fat. Foods such as legumes, nuts, seeds and milk contain a mixture of protein, fat and carbohydrate. There is absolutely no problem in the body's ability to digest such foods. The stomach will complain if it is overloaded or abused with alcohol or given excessive amounts of fat.

The stomach acts as a holding chamber for foods. Water empties quite quickly unless it contains glucose or any other type of sugar. For this reason, athletes who need to replace tissue losses as fast as possible should drink plain water.

When a mixture of nutrients is eaten, carbohydrates leaves the stomach first, protein follows and fats take the longest time to leave. This is why you tend to feel full for a long time after a fatty meal, and hungry soon after a Chinese meal which consists largely of rice and vegetables: mainly carbohydrate. When you eat a meal with plenty of carbohydrates, you feel full while the food is in the stomach. Such foods leave the stomach quite quickly and so the full feeling does not last for very long. Fatty foods such as sausages, chips or chocolates, may not be very filling (which means you can easily eat more than you need), but their high fat content means that they remain in the stomach for a longer period of time.

As food passes to the small intestine, the major part of digestion gets under way. Various enzymes which break down proteins, fats and carbohydrates are secreted into the intestine and convert each nutrient into its component parts. Fats are broken down to fatty acids and glycerol, proteins are digested to their component amino acids, and complex carbohydrates are converted to simple sugars such as glucose and fructose. Dietary fibre is separated from the nutrients and goes through to the large intestine where its digestion process is carried out by bacteria.

Foods which contain dietary fibre take a little longer to be digested because of the mechanical business of separating the fibre. For this reason, foods which are rich in dietary fibre slow down the initial process of digestion and allow a much more gradual series of reactions to occur. This is particularly important for the carbohydrates. Straight sugar or glucose is digested reasonably fast and passes quite quickly into the blood. When sugar enters the blood, the body produces the hormone insulin to enable the glucose to pass from the blood into the tissues. Once the liver has taken some glucose to store as glycogen, and the muscles have taken their fill, any excess glucose is converted to body fat. Excess protein or fat also end up as body fat.

Complex carbohydrates, and carbohydrate foods which contain dietary fibre, take longer in the initial stages of digestion and so do not provoke the same stimulus to the production of insulin. Rather than a rush of glucose, and the inevitable conversion of some to body fat, foods containing complex carbohydrate and dietary fibre provide a slower, steadier stream of glucose which is more likely to be used for energy.

The results of some studies have been used to cloud this issue. If isolated foods are eaten, and their effect on blood glucose is measured, we find that some foods produce a faster rise in the blood glucose than others. Carrots, for example, produce a reasonably sudden rise in blood sugar. This effect of particular foods on the blood glucose is described as the glycaemic index. It is sometimes used to justify sugar and discredit foods such as carrots. This is quite invalid and more recent studies have shown that when foods are eaten cooked, or eaten in combination with other foods, their glycaemic index may be different from when they are eaten separately. The issue of glycaemic index is not a sound basis on which to select foods.

It has also been found that the insulin response and the uptake of glucose by the tissues are largely affected by the amount of dietary fibre present in the food. With high-fibre foods, less insulin must be produced, and the uptake of glucose proceeds at a steady pace. Sudden rushes of glucose into the blood can thus be avoided by taking carbohydrates in a form with dietary fibre. Complex carbohydrate foods and fruits are the ideal ways to provide glucose to the tissues. By avoiding a sudden oversupply of glucose, we can also avoid excess production of body fat.

Why carbohydrates are regarded as fattening

Carbohydrates contribute just 16 kilojoules per gram. By comparison, proteins have 17 kilojoules gram, alcohol has 29 kilojoules per gram, while fats have a hefty 37 kilojoules per gram. So why are carbohydrates considered to be fattening?

There are two major reasons. The first concerns sugar. Like all carbohydrates, sugar has only 16 kilojoules per gram. However, sugar slips down so effortlessly that it is easy to take in huge quantities without even being aware of most of it! Sugar has thus given all carbohydrates a bad name.

The second reason why carbohydrates are thought to be fattening is that most slimming diets tell you so. Don't Eat Carbohydrates, The Carbohydrate-Counter's Diet, The Low-Carbohydrate Diet: there are hundreds of variations on this theme. These diets restrict carbohydrate to cause a large loss of water from the body. This shows up as a loss of weight on the scales and dieters believe that they are losing weight. The body's fat content is probably unchanged but the loss of water brings a sensation of instant success. Unfortunately, the water loss is temporary and the lost weight soon returns. Most slimmers then blame themselves or their metabolism for the regaining of the weight and remain totally ignorant that it was the foolish diet which was responsible for the temporary dehydration. As we shall see in chapter 11, these diets can actually make the would-be slimmer fatter. The unfortunate consequence of these diets has been a legacy of fear of carbohydrates.

If carbohydrates such as sugar or flour are combined with a lot of fat, as is the case with cakes, pastries, biscuits, chocolates and most icecreams, we can rightly tag them as fattening. If heaps of butter or margarine are piled onto foods such as bread or potatoes, their ultimate fate may well be fat too. It is not the carbohydrates which are at fault, but their accompanying *fat*. Complex carbohydrates alone are rarely fattening since they are so filling that their consumption is usually self-limiting.

Glycogen

Once complex carbohydrates are broken down, the glucose is taken by the blood to the muscles and the liver where it is converted to glycogen, a convenient storage form of glucose.

57

The glycogen in the liver is important to keep the glucose level in the blood constant. Most of the body's essential organs can use a mixture of glucose and fatty acids for fuel. The brain, however, can only run on glucose. The body therefore has a number of mechanisms to maintain the level of glucose in the blood to protect the brain.

The first effect of a drop in blood sugar level is a hunger pang. If you ignore this signal, you may have noticed that after a few minutes it goes away. This is because the body decides that no food is forthcoming and it had better break down some of its liver glycogen to replenish the blood sugar level. When this is used up, another hunger pang occurs, usually about 45 to 50 minutes after the first. If this too is ignored, more liver glycogen is broken down. Once the liver glycogen supply gets low, the body begins to break down some of its lean protein tissue to provide some glucose. Body fat cannot be converted to glucose.

The glycogen in the liver is also used during exercise. It is used as a fuel and also to keep the blood sugar level normal so that the brain can function properly. Fasting produces a sharp decline in the amount of glycogen in the liver. It is therefore undesirable to fast before any physical activity.

The glycogen in the muscles is used for both anaerobic and aerobic activities. For short, high-intensity anaerobic activities, such as sprinting, glycogen is the only fuel which is available to the muscle. For longer activities, the muscles can use both glucose (from glycogen) and fatty acids as fuel. The longer the glycogen supplies last, the more physical activity can be performed. Endurance activities thus depend on maximising the body's stores of glycogen.

If the diet contains plenty of carbohydrate, more glycogen can be supplied to the muscles to provide energy for physical activity. Stores of glycogen in the muscles are important both for endurance events and for high-intensity exercise.

If the diet lacks carbohydrate, glycogen in the muscles will not be replenished. Exercise then becomes difficult. Even though fatty acids are a source of fuel, fats cannot be completely burned for fuel if there is not some carbohydrate present. Thus the typical Western diet, with its low content of complex carbohydrate is more likely to produce a nation of spectator sportspeople than participants. It is hardly fair to expect people to exercise if they are consuming a diet which makes physical exertion difficult.

Those who need to lose weight should also note that more kilojoules are used up when the muscles have plenty of glycogen. Researchers have been able to show that depleting the muscles of glycogen resulted in only 50 per cent of the kilojoules being used compared with muscles containing plenty of glycogen. Most popular slimming diets reduce glycogen stores to a minimum (see chapter 11). With these diets, exercise is much less valuable in burning up kilojoules than occurs when the diet contains adequate amounts of carbohydrate.

Exercise itself leads to an increase in the capacity of the muscles to store glycogen. One group of researchers exercised one leg of their subjects to the point at which most of the glycogen was used up. They then allowed their subjects to rest for three days while eating a high-carbohydrate diet. Measurements of the glycogen stores in each leg showed that the leg which had been exercised stored twice the amount of glycogen as the leg which had not been exercised. Both legs had access to the same amount of glucose and hormones to make glycogen, but the exercised leg took up the most. The combination of physical activity *and* plenty of carbohydrate is the ideal way to maximise glycogen stores throughout the body's muscles (endurance events are discussed in chapter 12).

Simple carbohydrates (other than sugar)

Fruits, milk and yoghurt provide sugars including fructose and lactose. Fruits are good sources of dietary fibre and vitamins (particularly C and A), while milk and yoghurt are valuable for their calcium and riboflavin.

For peak performance, the diet should include both fruits and milk. In general, most adults should aim for at least three pieces of fruit a day and 500 millilitres of milk, preferably a low-fat variety.

How much carbohydrate for peak performance?

For those who have lots of physical activity, the exact amount of complex carbohydrate will depend on the ability to eat volumes of food. Some protein is needed, a very small amount of fat is essential, and the rest of the diet should consist of complex carbohydrate foods and fruit.

For a top athlete, at least 65 per cent of the diet should be carbohydrates with 45 to 50 per cent as complex carbohydrate and the rest as sugars. For those with lower levels of physical activity, it is ideal to have at least 60 per cent of the diet as carbohydrate. A greater percentage will do no harm, but the large quantities of food required can be a problem. The Pritikin diet has about 75 per cent of its kilojoules coming from complex carbohydrate, a level which is difficult for those requiring a high-kilojoule level to achieve since the stringent cutbacks in protein and fat mean many hours of crunching carbohydrates.

To achieve a level of 60 per cent carbohydrate in a diet, an 59 average man would need around 350 grams and a woman about 300 grams of carbohydrate a day. This will include complex carbohydrates, simple sugars found in fruit and milk, and sugar which has been added to foods. Appendix 1c gives appropriate levels for people at different weights and stages of physical activity.

The table below sets out the complex carbohydrates in various foods and also the sugars found naturally in fruits and milk. This may help you to make your choice of carbohydrate. If you can manage to eat more complex carbohydrate, instead of some fat, go right ahead.

Table 5.1 Complex carbohydrate in various foods

Food	Complex carbohydrate (grams)
Bread, wholemeal or white, thin slice	14
toast slice	16–18
Raisin bread, regular slice	16
Lebanese flatbread, large	60
Pita bread, average size	30
Muffin, each half	14
Crumpet, 1	18
Rye crispbread, 2	10
Wheat crispbread, 2	6–10
Weetabix, 2	22
Homemade muesli (see recipe, Appendix 1e)	27
Breakfast cereal, 30g	20
Porridge, cooked, 1 cup	25
Rice, cooked, 1 cup	30
Pasta, cooked, 1 cup	40
Potato, 125g	25
Most vegetables, average serve	5–6
Corn, 1 cup or 1 cob	25
Baked beans, 1 cup	40
Kidney, lima or other beans, 1 cup	40
Banana, average size	5
Meat, cheese, milk, chicken, fish	0

**Table 5.2 Simple carbohydrate in various foods (excluding sugar*)
— continued**

Food	Simple carbohydrate (grams)
Milk, regular or skim, 250mL	12
Shape	16
Hi-Lo or Rev	14
Buttermilk, 250mL	11
Flavoured milk contains an extra 10g of added sugar per 250mL	
Cottage cheese, 100g	0
Ricotta cheese, 100g	2

**Table 5.2 Simple carbohydrate in various foods (excluding sugar*)
— continued**

Food	Simple carbohydrate (grams)
Yoghurt, natural, 200g	13
low fat, natural, 200g	14
Flavoured yoghurt contains an extra 18g of added sugar per 200g	
Icecream, 150mL	3
Icecream also contains 13g of added sugar per 150mL	
Fruits	
Apple, medium	16
dried, 50g	38
Apricots, 2, average size	6
dried, 50g	22
Avocado, half	2
Banana, medium	17
Blackberries, 125g (half a punnet)	10
Cherries, 200g	20
Currants, dried, 30g	19
Custard apple, 100g	15
Dates, dried, 6	28
Figs, fresh, 1	5
dried, 50g	26
Grapes, 200g	28
Grapefruit, half, medium	4
Guava, average	3
Honeydew melon, 200g	16
Kiwi fruit, medium	9
Mandarin, medium	11
Mango, 1	24
Passionfruit, 1	3
Papaw, 200g	14
Peach, medium	10
Pear, medium	15
Pineapple, 200g	16
Prunes, 6, medium	24
Raisins, 30g	20
Raspberries, 125g (half a punnet)	7
Rhubarb, 1 cup, cooked	2
If stewed with sugar, add 25g of sugar	
Rockmelon, 200g	10
Strawberries, half a punnet	8
Sultanas, 30g	20
Watermelon, 200g	11

*Content of added sugar in various foods is covered in chapter 4.

Practical hints for eating more healthy carbohydrates

1   Rid yourself of the idea that complex carbohydrate foods are fattening. Until your attitude changes, it will be difficult for your eating habits to improve.

61

2 Eat very little fat so that you will have more 'room' for complex carbohydrates.

3 Choose a breakfast cereal which is mostly complex carbohydrate rather than one which has a large percentage of sugar (see Table 4.1).

4 Include thick slices of toast at breakfast.

5 Snack on bread, rolls, wholegrain crispbread, muffins, crumpets, vegetables, breakfast cereals (at any time of the day) and bananas.

6 Make lunch a healthy sandwich or have some potato, beans, pasta, rice or some other grain food.

7 Base your evening meal on rice, pasta, potatoes and vegetables and use meat as an accompaniment rather than as the star performer.

8 Choose fruit as a dessert or a snack between meals.

9 Add fruit to your breakfast cereal.

10 Make low-fat fruit shakes by blending low-fat milk with some ice cubes and fruits such as bananas, strawberries or melon.

For peak performance

- Complex carbohydrates plus the carbohydrate from fruits and milk should make up approximately 60 per cent of your daily diet. The appropriate quantities to provide this amount are listed in Appendix 1c.

- Glycogen stores can be increased by eating plenty of complex carbohydrate. Endurance athletes should aim for a high intake of complex carbohydrate at all times, rather than trying to carbohydrate load just before an event.

- Take care not to add too much fat of any type to bread, pasta, potatoes and other forms of complex carbohydrate. Peak performance needs plenty of carbohydrate, not fat.

- Remember that carbohydrates have the lowest kilojoule content (less than half the kilojoules of fat). They are unlikely to increase body fat levels unless eaten with a lot of fat.

6

Dietary fibre:
Are you getting enough?

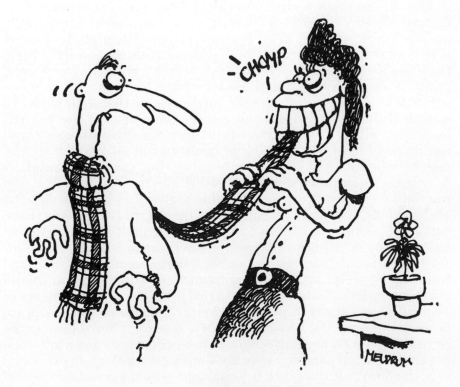

DIETARY fibre was forgotten for many years. With its obvious association with the intestine, it was simply not considered a polite topic of conversation. In recent years, a growing realisation of the value of dietary fibre has brought it out of hiding to resume its rightful place as an important part of the daily diet. Far from being just a good way to prevent constipation, nutritionists are discovering that dietary fibre has a number of other important roles.

Fibre fallacies

A number of notions relating to dietary fibre are false.

The first myth is that dietary fibre is one substance. Just as there are different vitamins, each with quite distinct actions in the body, so there are various forms of dietary fibre which have separate purposes. These are not yet fully understood but nutritionists are beginning to unravel the mysteries of the large intestine and discover what actually goes on in its murky depths.

The second myth is that unprocessed bran is synonymous with dietary fibre. Considering that it is a reasonably unpalatable product, sales of unprocessed bran are remarkably high. Its success is undoubtedly due to its ability to prevent constipation. However, that does not necessarily make it ideal. Bran is a good source of some types of dietary fibre, but is no substitute for some other more valuable kinds. Many regular bran eaters assume that their ability to munch through a bowl of bran insures them against the hazards associated with a low-fibre diet. It doesn't. Some people also abuse unprocessed bran by taking large quantities in an attempt to lose weight. Such efforts are not only futile, but can be harmful. A substance in unprocessed bran called phytic acid can 'tie up' minerals such as iron, calcium and zinc so that they are unable to be absorbed by the body. Small quantities of bran will not have sufficient phytic acid for this to be significant, but regularly taking half a cup or more over a long period can cause problems. If you suffer from constipation, one to two level tablespoons of unprocessed bran can be useful without being hazardous. However, you should also eat a variety of other grain or cereal products as well as plenty of vegetables and fruits to provide a better balance of fibre. Unprocessed bran is not the whole fibre story. It seems absurd to strip the bran and germ from a perfectly well-balanced wheat grain and then eat all the parts separately. Why not simply eat wholegrain products?

A third myth is that fibre is 'roughage' which goes in one end of the body and emerges, undigested, some time later from the other. By its very definition, dietary fibre is *not* digested by the enzymes in the digestive juices in the stomach and small intestine. But it certainly *does* undergo digestion by bacteria in the large intestine.

Rather than passing through us, much of the dietary fibre we eat is actually absorbed by the body. Recent research suggests that it is the products resulting from the digestion of certain types of dietary fibre which provide its greatest value.

Different types of dietary fibre

Dietary fibre exists only in the vegetable kingdom, in grains, breads and cereal products, vegetables, fruits, legumes, seeds and nuts. Animal foods have no dietary fibre.

The major categories of dietary fibre include:

Pectin: the type of dietary fibre found in apples, citrus peel (and marmalade), jams and fruits.

Cellulose: the 'stringy' fibre in vegetables and also found in grains and cereal foods, fruits, nuts and seeds.

Hemi–cellulose: actually a number of related substances found in cereals and cereal products (including white bread), vegetables, fruits, nuts and seeds.

Lignin: a 'woody' type of fibre found in cereal husks, root vegetables and pears.

Polysaccharides: carbohydrate-related substances which occur in foods such as legumes and grains.

Gums: found in oats and legumes.

Saponins: found in alfalfa, asparagus, chick peas, eggplant, kidney beans, mung beans, oats, peas, peanuts, soya beans, spinach and sunflower seeds.

Mucilages and gels: usually added as thickeners in processed foods.

Early measurements of fibre only identified 'crude fibre' which represented the cellulose present. It was not until more sophisticated measurements were possible that the other forms of dietary fibre were able to be measured. For this reason, old food tables which list only the crude fibre content of foods may grossly underestimate the true dietary fibre content.

The old idea of fibre being 'stringy' does not apply to most types of dietary fibre. Pectin, for example, is a fine white powder which readily absorbs water. The gums in oats also absorb water to form a viscous solution rather than being an obviously coarse fibre. Foods such as celery and lettuce, where you can easily see the strings of fibre do not contribute much dietary fibre at all. Other vegetables, legumes and grain products have much more total fibre.

Digestion of dietary fibre

The large bowel is where most of the digestion of dietary fibre occurs. An army of bacteria (good ones) sets to work on different

65

types of fibre and breaks them down, producing valuable chemical substances in the process. These substances, known as volatile fatty acids, are then absorbed and play a role in regulating the levels of glucose and cholesterol in the blood. The acids produced are acetic, propionic and butyric. They are absorbed directly through the wall of the bowel, providing nourishment to the cells of the bowel wall.

The types of dietary fibre which are soluble in water (pectin, gums, mucilages) are almost entirely digested by bacteria. These types of fibre produce more of the valuable volatile fatty acids. Rolled oats and legumes both contain a high percentage of gummy types of dietary fibre which are thoroughly digested and help to control levels of cholesterol and glucose in the blood. They are excellent products for sportspeople.

Lignin, a particularly coarse fibre, is hardly digested at all. Cellulose and the hemi-celluloses are digested to a varying extent, depending on your individual intestine and the time food remains in it.

The digestion of various types of fibre also depends on the amount present. If you have a very low intake of cellulose, for example, most of it is digested. With a higher content of cellulose, less is broken down by the bacteria.

The physical condition of some foods is also important. Coarse bran absorbs lots of water and will pass through the large intestine faster than finely ground bran. Coarse bran forms soft faeces; fine bran forms small hard ones.

What dietary fibre does

Populations who eat plenty of dietary fibre have a very low incidence of bowel cancer, diabetes, gallstones, heart disease, diverticular disease, obesity and constipation. Constipation is a direct result of a diet which is low in fibre and also lacks sufficient water. Most of the other conditions, however, are likely to be due to several factors, especially a high intake of fat. Foods which are high in dietary fibre are usually low in fat whereas those which are high in fat generally have little or no dietary fibre. It is therefore difficult to say whether it is the presence of fibre or the absence of fat which provides the greater benefit. It is probably both.

Prevention of constipation

Once food residues and dietary fibre enter the large intestine (or the large bowel), bacteria begin their task. The more dietary fibre present, the greater the number of bacteria. More than half of faecal bulk is made up of bacteria. So eating more wholegrain cereals, fruits and vegetables is nature's way of creating more bacteria which you later excrete.

Another function of the large intestine is to re–absorb water from its contents. If water is not being absorbed, loose watery faeces are passed, as occurs with diarrhoea. If there is not enough food residues in the large intestine, or insufficient water, water is absorbed and the faeces become hard, dry and difficult to pass, as occurs with constipation. In diagnosing constipation, the frequency with which faeces are passed is much less important than the consistency. A soft stool which can be passed without difficulty is desirable.

Dietary fibre initially slows down the rate at which food is digested. Once separated from the other food components, however, dietary fibre increases the rate at which the contents of the large intestine are emptied. Some types of fibre act like a sponge, soaking up water and forming softer faeces. When bacteria ferment and digest certain types of dietary fibre, they multiply by the million in the process.

Various bowel problems can occur if the level of dietary fibre is too low. Haemorrhoids can develop with straining to pass hard faeces. Small pockets can also develop in the large intestine which may become inflamed, resulting in the common condition of diverticulitis. Irritable bowel syndrome occurs when food residues pass through the intestine very quickly. This condition may occur because of sensitivity to some food ingredient or it may be a reaction to tension.

Back in the fifth century BC, Hippocrates recognised the importance of plenty of fibre and advised people to eat unsieved or coarse-grained bread to prevent constipation. It took many years before the medical profession generally promoted the idea that an increase in the total amount of dietary fibre could prevent constipation, haemorrhoids and diverticulitis. Many people with irritable bowel syndrome also benefit from a high-fibre diet since the fibre absorbs water from the contents of the large intestine.

Constipation and its related conditions are common in Western countries where many food processing methods specialise in stripping away most of the dietary fibre from foods such as cereals and fruits. The result is that many hundreds of millions of doses of laxatives are sold annually.

Laxatives may act by irritating the wall of the large intestine, or by stimulating the peristaltic movements of the intestine, or, in the case of faecal softeners, by increasing the water content of the faeces. Frequent use of laxatives can reduce the tone of the muscles in the bowel so that constipation becomes chronic.

Fibre supplements contribute various types of fibre. Isolated types of dietary fibre behave quite differently from the same type of fibre in foods where the effects are influenced by the amount and type of other nutrients present. When you eat an apple, the pectin present

67

acts differently from the same amount of pectin taken as a separate supplement. When high-fibre foods enter the stomach and small intestine, the fibre initially slows down the rate at which other nutrients are digested and absorbed. Taking a supplement of purified fibre misses this effect. Most dietary fibre supplements contain quite modest quantities of fibre. A recommended daily dose of some of the major brands would contribute as much dietary fibre as half a small banana, without the other nutrients and valuable carbohydrate which the banana supplies.

With the desire for extreme slenderness in women, fibre supplements have become even more popular, this time as a supposed aid to weight control. Foods rich in dietary fibre provide a natural obstacle to overeating. Fibre supplements do not necessarily have this advantage. The idea that taking fibre supplements will cause food to pass through the intestine too fast to contribute its kilojoules is rubbish. The inference that taking fibre supplements will make you slim may be profitable but it's not valid for effective weight control.

If we ate sufficient dietary fibre, constipation would be as rare as it is in countries where highly processed foods are not consumed. Laxatives and fibre supplements would be unnecessary. Drinking enough water and having regular exercise are also important to prevent constipation. Sportspeople should be especially diligent in drinking plenty of water. Sweating can cause a large loss of water from the body leaving insufficient for the large intestine. As some sportspeople have found, all they need to conquer constipation is more fluid.

Prevention of cancer of the colon and rectum

One of the major 'fathers' of fibre, Dr Denis Burkitt, put forward the theory that a low-fibre diet allowed cancer-causing substances to remain in contact with the wall of the bowel for a longer time, increasing the risk of abnormalities in the cells. Plenty of dietary fibre would dilute the concentration of any harmful chemicals and reduce their potency.

Cancers of the bowel are common in Western countries where the diet lacks dietary fibre. They are rare in countries where the staple diet has plenty of fibre. It is tempting to claim therefore that dietary fibre is protective against cancers of the colon and rectum. However, there are also other dietary differences which may play a role, especially involving fat. Whether fibre or fat is the most relevant factor in the development of bowel cancer is not yet fully understood. Current research suggests that it may be a joint effect.

Dietary fibre seems to protect against bowel cancer by one or more of the following mechanisms:

- it increases the contents of the bowel and so dilutes any cancer-causing chemical substances;
- it reduces the time potentially harmful chemical substances remain in contact with the bowel wall;
- it binds substances called bile acids which are believed to promote bowel cancer;
- it alters the bacteria in the bowel, allowing the 'good' bacteria to multiply. These bacteria will prevent bile acids being converted to cancer-producing substances; and
- it allows bacteria to produce volatile fatty acids which are anti–cancer agents.

Not all types of dietary fibre will have each of these actions. It would therefore be wise to consume a mixture of different types of dietary fibre for maximum protection. A low-fat diet would add at least as much, and perhaps even more, protection.

Control of blood cholesterol levels

The relationship between dietary fibre and cholesterol is not simple. Different types of fibre affect cholesterol in various ways. Saponins, for example, bind substances called bile acids. These chemicals are normally made from cholesterol in the body and they take part in the digestion of fats. If certain types of dietary fibre bind the bile acids so that they are unavailable, the body must convert even more cholesterol into bile acids. The end result is that the cholesterol is 'used up' in this way with less being available to clog up the arteries. Lignin, found in cereal fibre and root vegetables, may also bind bile acids and reduce cholesterol levels.

The water-soluble fibres found in pectin and the gummy fibres in oats and legumes also reduce blood cholesterol levels. Fruits, oats and legumes obviously have a lot going for them in the fibre stakes.

A diet high in dietary fibre is also likely to reduce the chances of gallstones. These stones are made from cholesterol which has been deposited out of its normal solution in the bile. Gallstones are common in those who are overweight and in those who consume a high proportion of the diet as fat.

Control of blood sugar levels

The body always tries to maintain a level of glucose in the blood within certain limits. This enables the brain and other vital organs to have a ready supply of energy. For anyone engaged in physical activity, some of the blood sugar can also be used as a source of fuel, especially in endurance events. High-fibre foods give a steadier release of energy over a longer period of time than quickly digested foods, such as sugar.

69

Once again, it is difficult to know where to lay the credit. A diet which is high in dietary fibre will also contain a higher content of complex carbohydrate. Is it this carbohydrate, or is it the fibre, or are both involved in the control of blood sugar levels? Tests seem to indicate that both may be involved. In nature, most carbohydrates occur with dietary fibre. It is only in highly processed foods such as sugar, refined cereals or fruit juices that we have the opportunity to eat carbohydrate without its protective fibre.

In some people, especially diabetics, blood sugar levels can fluctuate. A high-fibre diet seems to improve control of blood sugar levels, with pectin (from fruit) and the gummy fibres in oats and legumes being the important types. Diabetics can often lower their dose of insulin or other drugs if the dietary fibre content of their daily meals and snacks is increased. As a bonus, a high-fibre diet decreases levels of blood fats.

Guar gum, a type of dietary fibre which can be extracted from certain plants and legumes, also seems to be beneficial in controlling blood sugar levels.

Appetite and weight control

Since foods containing fibre are filling, dietary fibre is a natural obstacle to overeating. A bowl of porridge eaten before leaving home in the morning, for example, is filling enough to reduce the chances of buying a doughnut on the way to work. Many people confuse filling with fattening and deliberately shun foods such as rolled oats or potatoes because they fear that they will make them fat. In fact, a potato has fewer kilojoules than a glass of orange juice. Eating plenty of fibre-rich foods makes it easier to control body weight.

Hunger rumbles begin when the blood sugar level drops. Foods which are high in sugar but low in fibre sometimes produce a surge in blood sugar levels followed by a sudden fall. On the other hand, foods which are high in dietary fibre are digested more slowly than refined products and do not produce rapid rises and falls in blood sugar levels. Eating a good hearty wholemeal bread sandwich (or two) for lunch will give a steadier release of energy during the afternoon than a quickly munched chocolate bar.

How much dietary fibre?

The typical Western diet has only about 15 grams of dietary fibre a day. People living in more primitive rural communities may eat five to six times this much.

Most nutritionists recommend a daily total of 30 to 40 grams of fibre. For those who are eating large quantities of food to provide sufficient energy for endurance activities, a higher daily total will be almost unavoidable if sufficient complex carbohydrate foods are being included since most sources of complex carbohydrate are also good sources of dietary fibre.

The problem of too much fibre occasionally occurs with athletes who are eating very large quantities of food such as wholegrain breads and cereals. The total fibre content may be so high that there is too much bulk to be eliminated.

Flatulence

When dietary fibre is increased, there will be a greater production of 'wind'. This is quite normal but can be socially embarrassing. Some people actually study this subject and their tests have shown that most people pass similar quantities of wind, but their perceptions of the amount vary considerably.

Whenever the fibre content of the diet is being increased, it should be done gradually. Sudden changes are too much for the intestine and greater quantities of gas will be produced. It is also important to chew foods thoroughly before swallowing.

Beans are notorious for producing flatulence. The amount of gas produced after eating beans or peas is much greater if the legumes have been dehusked. For example, chick pea powder with the husks removed produces much more flatulence than normal chick peas. It is thought that the husk binds some minerals, such as iron or manganese, which are required for the formation of gas. The moral of this is that you should eat beans and peas with their transparent-looking 'skins' on. Many people also find that rinsing dried beans or peas before cooking eliminates some of the flatulence that comes after eating them.

Where to find dietary fibre

Use the table below to check out the fibre content of your daily diet. You should be aiming for at least 30 to 40 grams.

Table 6.1 Dietary fibre content of foods

Food	Dietary fibre content (grams)
Breads	
Bread, average slice	2.5
white	0.6
toast thickness	0.9
high-fibre, white	1.8
multigrain	2.0
wholemeal	2.4
fruit loaf	1.0
Bread roll, white	1.4
wholemeal	5.1

71

Table 6.1   Dietary fibre content of foods — continued

Food	Dietary fibre content (grams)
Muffin, each half	1.2
Rye crispbread, 2	2.3
Crackerbread, wholemeal, 2	1.2
Breakfast cereals, grains / cereals, average serve	
Porridge	5.0
Weetabix, 2	2.8
Allbran	9.5
Bran Flakes	7.0
Cornflakes, Special K	negligible
Muesli	8.0
Muesli Flakes	3.6
Nutrigrain, Rice Bubbles	negligible
Unprocessed bran, 1 tablespoon	3.0
Wheatgerm, 1 tablespoon	2.0
Rice, white, 1 cup cooked	1.4
brown, 1 cup	2.8
Pasta, average serve	3.5
Cracked wheat, average serve	6.5
Vegetables, average serve	
Asparagus	1.5
Beans, green	3.0
kidney, soya, canned baked	9.5
Beansprouts	0.5
Broccoli	4.0
Brussels sprouts	3.0
Cabbage	2.0
Carrots	3.0
Cauliflower	2.0
Celery	1.0
Corn, 1 cob	6.5
Cucumber	0.2
Lentils	7.5
Lettuce	1.0
Mushrooms	2.5
Parsnip	3.0
Peas	7.5
Potato, with skin	5.5
peeled	1.5
Pumpkin	1.5
Spinach	4.5
Sweet potato	2.5
Tomato	2.0
Yam	4.0
Zucchini	2.0
Fruits	
Apple, 1, with skin	3.3
Apricots, 100g	2.0

Table 6.1 Dietary fibre content of foods — continued

Food	Dietary fibre content (grams)
Avocado, half	2.0
Banana, average	4.0
Blackberries, half a punnet	9.0
Cherries, 150g	2.5
Figs, fresh, 1	2.5
dried, 50g	9.0
Grapes, 200g	1.8
Grapefruit, half	2.0
Kiwi fruit, average	2.2
Mango, 1	3.5
Melon, 200g	2.0
Nectarine, 1 large or 2 small	2.5
Orange, average	3.0
Passionfruit, 2, average	6.5
Papaw, 150g	3.5
Peach, average	1.8
Pear, average	3.5
Pineapple, average slice	2.1
Plums, 2	3.2
Prunes, 6, medium	8.0
Raisins or sultanas, 50g	3.5
Raspberries, half a punnet	9.3
Rhubarb, cooked, average serve	4.0
Strawberries, half a punnet	2.8
Nuts and seeds	
Almonds, 30g	4.3
Brazil nuts, 30g	2.7
Cashews, 30g	2.4
Coconut, fresh, 75g	10.0
dried, 15g	3.5
Hazelnuts, 30g	1.8
Macadamia nuts, 30g	2.0
Peanuts, 30g	2.4
Peanut butter, average spread	3.0
Pecan nuts, 30g	2.5
Pine nuts, 30g	2.0
Walnuts, 30g	1.6
Pepitas (pumpkin seeds), 30g	3.0
Sesame seeds, 5g	1.3
Sunflower seeds, 20g	3.3
Others	
Popped corn, 1 cup	1.0
Corn chips, small packet	0.5
Meats of all types, poultry, seafoods	0
Milk, cheese, dairy products	0
Eggs	0
Fats	0
Sugars	0

Practical hints to increase your fibre intake

1   Begin the day with a plate of rolled oats or other wholegrain cereal, topped with a tablespoon each of wheatgerm and unprocessed bran.
2   Try to choose wholegrain products wherever possible, for example: brown rice, wholemeal bread (preferably with added wholegrains) or wholegrain breakfast cereals.
3   Don't forget the beans. Whether they're canned or home-cooked, they are all excellent sources of dietary fibre.
4   Eat fruit rather than drinking the juice.
5   Nibble on carrots or other vegetables, or dried fruits.
6   Choose fruit, wholerye crispbread, wholemeal bread or toast as snack foods.
7   Have a vegetarian main meal sometimes. All dried beans, peas and lentils are excellent sources of dietary fibre.
8   Try some new products such as buckwheat, rolled rye, millet, or cornmeal (also sold as polenta).
9   Look for some cracked wheat (also known as burghul). It is quickly prepared by covering with boiling water and leaving to stand with the lid on for five to ten minutes.
10   Eat more potatoes, preferably steamed, microwaved or baked in their jackets.
11   Make vegetables the major part of your evening meal, with meat as a sideline rather than as the star performer.

For peak performance

- Make sure your diet contains 40 grams of dietary fibre a day. Larger quantities may be unavoidable for endurance athletes who are eating a lot of carbohydrate foods. If you find that you are excreting too much bulk, substitute some white bread for the wholegrain varieties, choose white rice and restrict fruit to about four pieces a day.
- If you suffer from constipation, remember it is not only caused by a lack of dietary fibre, but also by a deficiency of water.
- Restrict unprocessed bran to two tablespoons a day. Large quantities may interfere with the absorption of important minerals such as iron, zinc and calcium.

7

Alcohol:
How to handle it

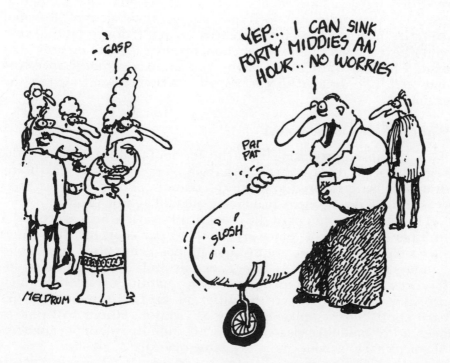

ALCOHOL can be one of life's social pleasures. It can also cause more havoc to health than almost anything else we eat or drink. In small quantities alcohol appears to be harmless and some studies have shown that moderate drinkers actually live longer than teetotallers. Whether this is due to the beneficial effects small quantities of alcohol have on blood fats or to its relaxing effects is not known.

But before you reach gleefully for your favourite tipple, you should know that studies showing harmful effects of alcohol far outnumber those praising its virtues. Unfortunately, any good effects are restricted to consuming small quantities of alcohol.

We do not always imbibe small quantities of alcohol. Each year we down around 5 litres of spirits, over 200 glasses of wine and over 100 litres of beer: an average of more than one drink per day for every person in the country. When you consider that many people drink no alcohol at all, the rest of the population must be a very thirsty lot.

Alcoholic beverages have been important to humans for as long as recorded history. One theory even proposes that the accidental discovery that grains would ferment to produce alcohol provided primitive man with the first incentive to settle down. Noting that wild wheat and barley and water could produce a bubbling brew that made whoever drank it feel happy, our hunter–gatherer ancestors may well have decided that a nomadic existence went against the grain.

What it is and what it does

Alcohol can be produced from the fermentation of grains, fruits vegetables, sugars or even the sap from trees. Almost any carbohydrate can be fermented to produce ethanol. The process occurs as yeasts break down sugars producing alcohol as a by-product.

The alcoholic content of different drinks varies. Beer is around 4 to 5 per cent alcohol, wines are 10 to 15 per cent, fortified wines such as sherry or port are around 20 per cent, while spirits and liqueurs may be as high as 40 per cent alcohol. In spite of these differences, there seems to be a certain quantity of alcohol which provokes a specific effect: the different sizes of 'standard' drinks each contribute a similar quantity of alcohol. Thus a half pint of beer, a 125–millilitre glass of wine, a 60–millilitre tot of port or a nip of spirits each provide about the same quantity of alcohol.

Alcohol is both a drug and a food. As a drug it acts on the central nervous system which controls most of our actions, thoughts and emotions. Its numbing qualities were once used medically as an anaesthetic but, in milder doses, alcohol creates a sense of well-being and relaxation. Contrary to popular belief, alcohol is not a stimulant

76

but acts as a depressant, slowing down the processes occurring in the brain.

As a food, alcohol is somewhat different from other nutrients because it is absorbed directly into the bloodstream through the walls of the stomach and the small intestine. Unlike other nutrients, it requires no digestion. Each gram of alcohol has 29 kilojoules (7 Calories), but contributes no vitamins, minerals or proteins.

What happens after drinking?

Some alcohol is absorbed from the stomach (this is especially the case with sparkling wines, champagne, or spirits mixed with anything fizzy) and the rest enters the small intestine. Since it needs no digestion, alcohol is rapidly absorbed straight through the intestinal walls into the blood.

If there is food in the stomach, it will take longer for the total contents of the stomach to pass into the small intestine slowing the rate at which alcohol is absorbed into the blood. Conversely, drinking on an empty stomach produces a rapid absorption of alcohol into the blood. Bubbles (as in champagne or carbonated drinks) cause rapid emptying of the stomach so that alcohol enters the small intestine and then the bloodstream very quickly. Whisky–and–soda thus causes a more rapid rise in blood alcohol than straight whisky. A champagne cocktail will have the greatest impact of all, especially if presented to an empty stomach.

The peak concentration of alcohol is usually reached 20 to 30 minutes after finishing a drink. If you have eaten at the same time (or just before), it will take about 30 to 60 minutes longer before alcohol enters the blood.

Once alcohol leaves the small intestine, it goes into the blood and is taken via the liver to be distributed by the blood to the body cells. Blood is constantly circulated throughout the body and each time it passes through the liver, a small portion of alcohol is removed and converted to carbon dioxide which is later breathed out.

Only about 8 to 10 grams of alcohol can be broken down each hour. This is equal to the alcohol content of a standard drink (a middy of beer, a nip of spirits, a glass of wine). If you have a beer before dinner, half a bottle of wine with dinner and a port to follow, it will take about five hours after you have finished the evening's drinking for the liver to remove the alcohol from the blood. The liver does not even begin to remove alcohol until after the maximum concentration has been passed. There is no way to speed up the process. Some people metabolise alcohol at an even slower rate than the times quoted here.

The concentration of alcohol in the blood depends on a number of factors. The bigger and leaner your body, the lower the resulting concentration of alcohol in your blood from each drink. This response is due to the amount of water in the body. Muscle has a high water content while fat contains little water. Since the alcohol distributes itself throughout the body's water, lean people with a higher percentage of muscle, and hence a higher water content, will have a lower concentration of alcohol in their blood. For this reason, lean muscular people may be less affected by alcohol than those who are smaller or fatter. For example, a lean fit person weighing 80 kilograms will have a much lower blood alcohol concentration after a given amount of alcohol than someone of the same weight who has more body fat. Most women have a higher body fat level and will have a higher blood alcohol reading than males of the same weight. If we follow this to its extreme, a small, well-rounded woman would be foolish to drink champagne cocktails on an empty stomach and then attempt to drive!

After the drinking is over

The initial effects of alcohol include a feeling of relaxation. This may be followed by a feeling of animation and talkativeness as you become less inhibited and more self–confident. As the brain and nervous system become affected by the alcohol, there is a loss of judgement, and tasks requiring coordination become difficult. Driving becomes dangerous.

A feature of such effects may be the denial that they exist. Alcohol also increases aggressive behaviour and most people affected by alcohol do not know that they are so affected. Drivers who have been drinking may drive in an aggressive, risk-taking manner, quite unaware of their crazy actions.

As the concentration of alcohol increases further, reaction times slow down, speech may become blurred, nausea is a distinct possibility and desire for sleep may become overwhelming. Some people become more aggressive, angry or emotional. If drinking continues, loss of coordination increases to the point where walking becomes impossible and vomiting, stupor or even a coma may occur.

The hangover

Most people stop drinking before too many symptoms develop. Even so they may have to endure a hangover as the body undergoes withdrawal symptoms while ridding itself of the alcohol. Symptoms include headache, dizziness and nausea. Most sufferers are intensely sensitive to light and sound as their nervous system recovers from the depressing effects of alcohol. Alcohol affects the kidney hormones which control water loss from the body. The dry mouth and the headache are partly due to dehydration.

Alcohol also enlarges blood vessels in the brain, contributing to the morning-after headache. Some other types of alcohol in some beverages may also cause headaches. A few people develop headaches because of a sensitivity to the amines present in wines made from Shiraz grapes.

The nausea which may accompany a hangover is due to the effects of alcohol on the brain and to the directly irritating effects of alcohol on the lining of the stomach. The liver is also so busy metabolising the alcohol that it may neglect its usual duties. Eating something, especially carbohydrates, will help nausea pass.

In general, the way to minimise alcohol concentration in the blood, and hence avoid the hangover, is to eat some food *before* drinking (preferably carbohydrate), have plenty of water (before, during and after drinking), drink slowly and preferably drink less. Once alcohol is in the bloodstream, it is metabolised at a constant rate and time is the best medicine to rid the body of its effects. It takes hours for the body to remove alcohol and you may still be above legal limits of blood alcohol the next morning. If you're after peak performance, the best cure for a hangover is to avoid drinking enough to cause it!

The good news about alcohol

In small doses, alcohol can cheer you up, stimulate the appetite (which may or may not be a good thing), help control blood pressure and create social goodwill. Small quantities of alcohol may even be a help in keeping blood fats normal.

Studies which have shown that moderate drinkers have a longer life expectancy than total abstainers put the benefits down to the effect alcohol has on the coronary arteries. In small doses, alcohol dilates these arteries, relieving pressure on the heart. Too much and it begins to work like a poison on the heart muscle.

The list of benefits from alcohol is short and most are wiped out if the dose goes too high. Blood pressure and blood fats are particularly likely to turn against you if you drink very much.

The bad news about alcohol

Apart from generally making you feel bad the morning after, regular heavy drinking can produce permanent damage to the body. Many people, particularly some men, boast about their drinking prowess; some even judge their 'manhood' by the amount they can drink. Some pretend that alcohol has no harmful effects on a 'real' man; most probably prefer not to think too much about the effects of alcohol.

79

Australians hold thirteenth place in the world for alcohol consumption and fourth ranking for beer swilling. While this is a source of pride for many Australians, it is a more sobering thought that alcohol probably causes more health, social and economic problems than any other substance. It has been estimated that one in 25 people working in industry has an alcohol problem with associated costs of over $1 billion a year. On a personal level, more than 1.3 million people have social or health problems due to alcohol.

There are hundreds of thousands of people officially classified as alcoholics and many more who are not in any national statistics. The real figure is thought to be much higher. It is a popular misconception that alcoholics are 'down-and-outers'. Many are found in the ranks of apparently successful business people. Most deny their condition.

Alcohol is a factor in more than 40 per cent of all road accidents. It is also involved in 50 per cent of drownings and in many domestic accidents.

Too much alcohol damages the liver, the pancreas, the heart and the brain. The liver becomes scarred and fibrous and can no longer perform its usual roles. Damage to the liver may take 10 to 20 years to develop. The first sign may be a swollen liver. This is followed by nausea, pain, bruising or a jaundiced appearance. The liver loses its soft resilience and becomes a shrivelled hard lump. The final outcome is liver failure and death. Cirrhosis of the liver is one of the major causes of death in Australian men between the ages of 25 and 65. It is generally associated with frequent drinking rather than with drunkenness.

Brain cells are also damaged by alcohol. Medical experts can easily pick a six-to-eight-drink-a-day-man by looking at a picture of his brain. Put simply, if you drink too much, your brain will shrink. Bouts of heavy drinking are especially likely to knock out a significant number of brain cells. Even six drinks a day will destroy a significant number of brain cells. Australia has the dubious distinction of having the highest rate of alcohol-related brain damage in the world.

Alcohol can also increase the levels of triglycerides. These fats circulate in the blood and cause heart disease. Alcohol can also affect various hormones of the adrenal cortex in the kidney allowing blood pressure to rise. A relatively modest intake of three to four drinks a day can also increase blood pressure, although smaller quantities may actually reduce it.

There are other problems too. Cancer of the oesophagus (the tube leading to the stomach) is 25 times more common among heavy drinkers than among light drinkers. Beer is also implicated in the development of bowel cancer. Both beer and whisky contain a nitrosamine substance which can stimulate the growth of cancerous cells.

Those who believe that alcohol is an aphrodisiac are also in for some disappointment. Shakespeare penned the immortal line 'it provokes and it unprovokes; it provokes the desire, but it takes away the performance . . .'. Since those times, it has been shown that alcohol causes the liver to produce an enzyme which destroys the male sex hormone, testosterone. The result: a loss of potency. Males who are heavy drinkers can look forward to a shrinkage of the testicles. Women are not immune to the effects of alcohol either. Too much causes the ovaries to shrink and periods to stop.

Alcohol also uses up the body's stores of thiamin (vitamin B_1). Heavy drinkers can develop a disease known as Wernicke–Korsakoff syndrome in which they experience abnormal memory, eye defects and trembling. These symptoms can be reversed by giving thiamin and it is sometimes suggested that this vitamin should be added to beer.

And last, but by no means least, alcohol is a potent source of kilojoules. As such it must accept a share of the blame for many of those people who are overweight.

How much?

After such a list of problems, you may be tempted to join the ranks of the teetotallers. However, medical evidence does not suggest that this is necessary. As mentioned earlier, light drinkers tend to live longer than total abstainers.

The secret to healthy drinking lies with appropriate quantities. Early recommendations were for an upper daily limit for males of 60 to 80 grams of alcohol, the amount in six to eight standard drinks. Medical authorities now consider this is too high and recommend a maximum level of three drinks (30 grams of alcohol) a day for women and six drinks (60 grams of alcohol) for men. For those who are carrying any excess flesh, these quantities should be reduced as far as is socially acceptable. One or two drinks a day would be a maximum.

For those involved in social eating and drinking at lunch and dinner, and wanting their bodies to keep functioning for peak performance, there is little choice but to drink less. Many business people have reached this conclusion and it is now quite common for alcohol not to be served at lunches.

For those who have some drinks before, during and after dinner, it is easy to overstep safe quantities of alcohol. Even if you have wisely decided not to drive after such an evening, that quantity of alcohol has the potential to harm the liver, the brain, to increase blood pressure and to increase risks of cancer.

The effects of drinking

The way you feel after alcohol can be described as follows :

Initial reaction:
- dashing/debonair
- dangerous/devilish
- dizzy/disturbed

Increasing consumption:
- disoriented/drunk
- dead drunk
- dead

Women and alcohol

Women are at a disadvantage: a smaller amount of alcohol will produce more adverse effects than with men. Women who are tall and have a larger frame and those who have sufficient physical activity to build up a large muscle mass will be less affected by alcohol.

There is also some variation in the intoxicating effects of alcohol at different times of the menstrual cycle. As most women know, sometimes they can have a couple of glasses of wine and feel no effects, while on other occasions the same quantity of alcohol will make it difficult to walk in a straight line. Women experience a stronger intoxicating effect of alcohol just before and just after their periods.

During pregnancy, alcohol crosses the placenta quite freely. Medical research has shown that women who drink heavily during pregnancy are more likely to have children with delayed learning ability, abnormalities of the joints and heart and possible structural abnormalities. Most of the research has looked at the effects of heavy drinking. However, there is some evidence that even a moderate consumption of two drinks a day during pregnancy may increase the risk of learning difficulties in the child. With present knowledge, there is no safe quantity of alcohol during pregnancy. For peak pregnancy performance, it is therefore wise for pregnant women to avoid all alcoholic drinks.

Alcohol and other drugs

Many drugs can increase the adverse effects of alcohol. Some anti–infective drugs slow down the rate at which alcohol can be metabolised by the liver. Other drugs may increase the rate at which alcohol is absorbed. Conversely, alcohol may increase the potency of some drugs.

Sleeping tablets can slow down the rate at which alcohol is used by the body. If you had been out drinking during the evening, arrived home and taken a sleeping tablet, you may well find that you are still over the legal blood alcohol concentration the next morning. Some antihistamines also interact with alcohol while the combination of alcohol and marihuana has been found to increase driving impairment.

Not all drugs interact with alcohol. However, it is wise if taking any form of medication to check with your doctor and/or pharmacist about possible interactions.

Myths about alcohol

An antidote to alcohol? There has been a long search for a magic formula which would allow us to drink and enjoy the effects of the alcohol, while freeing us from the problems of too much alcohol in the blood. The wonder product continues to elude us, although exorbitant claims have been made for various vitamins and particular foods.

Fructose or fruit sugar has been touted as an aid to instant sobriety. Fructose does decrease the rate at which alcohol is absorbed into the blood, but only to a modest extent. Taking fructose is much the same as eating a meal while you are drinking. It helps but doesn't cancel out the alcohol. Very large quantities of fructose are not the answer as they produce stomach pains and vomiting. The cure may be worse than the complaint! Fructose solutions are also undesirable for diabetics, and their frequent use may cause liver damage. The greatest advantage in taking fructose probably lies in its distributor's bank balance. There's little point in wasting your money eating the stuff.

Coffee is frequently drunk before taking to the road. The caffeine in coffee may keep you awake but it does absolutely nothing to alter the alcohol content in the blood. It has no sobering effect and simply produces an awake drunk.

Vitamins B and C have been promoted as cures for too much drinking. Alcohol certainly depletes the body of some of the B-complex vitamins and is responsible for some of the brain disorders which accompany chronic heavy drinking. However, taking a vitamin pill will have no effect in getting rid of alcohol from the body.

A good physical workout is sometimes promoted for ridding the body of alcohol. The major effect of such action is that the workout will be at a lower level than normal. Alcohol and physical exertion do not mix. The kilojoules from alcohol are not available to the muscles until the alcohol has been metabolised. Exercise will not make you any more sober than sleeping will.

Alcohol acts as an aphrodisiac? Many foods and drinks are credited with increasing sexual desire. Alcohol does have an initial ability to increase self-confidence and reduce inhibitions, but large quantities of alcohol can hinder arousal and orgasm.

Alcohol warms the body? Once again, the popular belief is incorrect. Alcohol increases the loss of heat from body and should *not* be given to anyone with hypothermia.

A good tot of rum cures a cold? Sadly, this one is also a myth. The rum may make you less aware of the symptoms of a cold, but it has no effect on the condition.

Alcohol relieves tension? Initially this statement is true. However, using alcohol as a means of dealing with unresolved tension can lead to problem drinking and does nothing to help you cope with real problems.

Do you have an alcohol problem?

Ask yourself the following questions. If you answer 'yes' to several of them, you may need to reconsider your drinking habits.

1   Do you often find yourself thinking about your next drink?
2   Do you toss down a drink quickly?
3   Do you drink more when you feel you need to relax?
4   Do you often drink alone?
5   Do you ever hide alcoholic drinks?
6   Do you feel you're more of a social success once you've had a couple of drinks?
7   Do you drink before guests arrive?
8   Do you try to be nice to people to make up for anything you may have said or done while drinking?
9   Do you reward yourself with a drink after a hard day?
10   Has anyone ever suggested that you drink too much?
11   Do you become argumentative after a few drinks?
12   Do you need someone to get you home after you've been out drinking?

A few facts about drinks

Table 7.1   Alcohol content of drinks

Drink	Alcohol content	Kilojoules
Beer, can	18g	650 (155 Cals)
middy	14g	500 (120 Cals)
Light beer, (3%), can	11g	430 (105 Cals)
(2%), can	7g	380 (90 Cals)
Special light (0.9%), can	3g	300 (70 Cals)
Stout, middy		610 (145 Cals)

Table 7.1   Alcohol content of drinks — continued

Drink	Alcohol content	Kilojoules
Campari, 30mL		290 (70 Cals)
Champagne, 125mL		370 (90 Cals)
Cider, alcoholic, 250mL		360 (85 Cals)
Liqueurs, 20mL		250 (60 Cals)
Ouzo, 30mL		290 (70 Cals)
Pimms, 30mL	6g	290 (70 Cals)
Port, 60mL	11g	395 (95 Cals)
Sherry, dry, 60mL	11g	290 (70 Cals)
sweet or cream, 60mL	11g	370 (90 Cals)
Spirits (brandy, gin, rum, whisky, vodka)**		
single (30mL)	12g	290 (70 Cals)
double (60mL)	24g	580 (140 Cals)
Vermouth, dry, 60mL		290 (70 Cals)
sweet		370 (90 Cals)
Wine, 125mL*		
red or white	15g	350 (85 Cals)

*If used in cooking, the alcohol evaporates and virtually no kilojoules are contributed.
**If adding dry ginger ale, add on 240kJ (60 Cals) for every 200mL.
   If adding tonic, add on 300kJ (70 Cals) for every 200mL.
   If adding cola, add on 355kJ (85 Cals) for every 200mL.
   Soda water and mineral water have no kilojoules.

Practical hints to avoid too much alcohol

1   Drink a large glass of water or mineral water before starting on alcohol. This allows you to sip your alcoholic drink and make it last longer than if you down it to quench your thirst.
2   Drink slowly. You are not socially obliged to refill your glass while it is still full!
3   Try to avoid the practice of shouting rounds of drinks.
4   Make a positive decision about how many drinks you will have and stick to it.
5   Ask waiters not to refill your wine glass so that you can tell more accurately how much you have had.
6   Make sure you eat before and while your are drinking alcohol. This will slow down the rate at which alcohol is absorbed into the blood.
7   Ask for some soft drinks or iced water to be available so that you can drink less alcohol.

For peak performance

- Restrict alcoholic drinks as much as possible. One or two drinks a day will generally do no harm.
- For those engaged in strenuous physical activity, avoid alcohol before any event.

8

Protein:
Animal or vegetable?

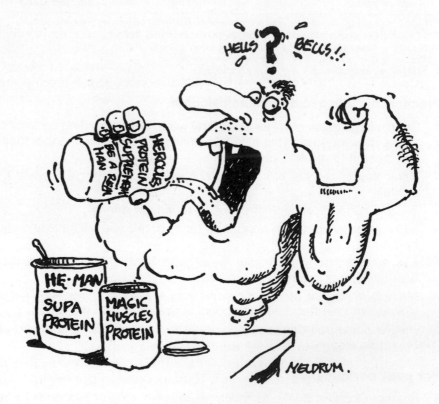

FOR many years, protein foods enjoyed 'motherhood' status. The very word protein means 'of first importance' and animal protein foods were certainly afforded that position. Protein will always be important as it is a vital part of every cell in the body but there is no valid reason for the excessive enthusiasm exhibited for animal protein foods. Many of these are high in fat and giving them prominence means that a high-protein diet may, inadvertently, be a high-fat diet.

Protein: why you need it

Too much protein is unnecessary but you do need some. All body cells contain protein. It is found in muscles, in organs such as the heart, liver and kidneys, in blood cells, in skin, hair and nails and in teeth and bones. Whenever growth is occurring, new cells are forming and protein requirements are increased. A child requires a higher percentage of protein than an adult. Protein needs also increase during pregnancy to provide for the needs of the growing baby.

Once growth stops, protein is still needed to replace cells which are lost through the wear and tear of normal living. Protein is also used by the body to make the enzymes which control the body's chemistry, the antibodies which fight infection, the haemoglobin (the material which carries oxygen in the blood), and certain hormones such as insulin.

Proteins and muscles

Some body builders almost worship protein, believing that an ample supply will produce the biceps and triceps they desire. It won't. Muscles do contain protein but that does not mean that stuffing yourself with extra quantities of protein will enlarge them. Muscles develop when they are used, and the ideal fuel for the use of muscles is complex carbohydrate, not protein.

Weight training is an ideal way to increase muscle mass. If you do not eat sufficient carbohydrate during weight training, the body may break down muscle to use as a source of fuel. A pattern of weight training combined with eating little carbohydrate can result in muscle being broken down rather than built up. This obviously defeats the whole purpose of weight training.

Growth of muscles requires protein, but the quantities for this are quite modest and are already likely to be present in the normal diet. Ordinary physical activity does not increase protein requirements much at all since the muscles use carbohydrate or fat as fuel in preference to protein. Taking extra protein in the form of amino acid or special protein supplements will not produce extra muscle growth.

Those involved in endurance events need more protein than sedentary people, as there is extra wear and tear on body tissues (including muscle fibres) during long arduous training. However, the extra quantities of protein are easily provided by a normal diet. Protein supplements are unnecessary except at times when there is massive tissue rebuilding such as that which occurs after severe burns which damage much of the body's tissues and skin area.

What about excess?

The fashion for high-protein diets has been blamed for the development of big beefy people. Early puberty may also be partly related to eating very large quantities of protein.

Protein's greatest problem concerns the company it keeps. Slabs of steak, hamburger mince, hearty helpings of meats in stews, cheeses, and breakfasts of sausages, bacon and eggs will contribute lots of protein but also stacks of saturated fats.

Animal protein foods also suffer from a total lack of dietary fibre. Since fibre is filling, a high-protein, low-fibre diet can easily deceive the appetite control mechanism so that you eat too much. Vegetable sources of protein, such as grains and legumes, have plenty of dietary fibre and thus are less likely to be overconsumed.

Once the body has met its protein requirements, any excess protein is converted to flabby body fat. If you eat steaks which hang over the edge of the plate, you are likely to find that before long, your stomach hangs over your belt. Some protein can be used for energy, but the body prefers to use carbohydrates or fats.

Eating a lot of protein also decreases the amount of calcium absorbed. Doubling the protein intake from 50 to 100 grams a day almost halves the amount of calcium which is absorbed.

Amino acids

Proteins are made up of smaller units called amino acids. When we eat foods, we digest their proteins and break them down to their separate amino acids. Our own body proteins are then synthesised from the appropriate amino acids. Foods contain a mixture of 23 amino acids. Provided the total amino acid pool is sufficient, most of our amino acids can be made in the body. However, eight known as essential amino acids, must be supplied from the food we eat.

Animal versus vegetable protein

Animal protein foods such as meats, fish, eggs, milk, yoghurt and cheese happen to contain all the essential amino acids. Vegetable
protein foods generally run low in one or two. However, combina-

tions of vegetable foods can easily supply the entire range of amino acids, including the essential amino acids.

Eggs have the best available selection of amino acids and these are easily assimilated into the human body. This makes eggs a convenient food, although by no means essential for body builders. The idea that eggs or other animal foods will provide a superior source of protein is totally invalid if a variety of vegetable foods is eaten. Recent research suggests that the foods need not be eaten even at the same meal but may be consumed several hours apart.

Vegetarians rarely have a problem obtaining sufficient protein. However, anyone who tries to live on a very restricted diet, such as fruitarians (who eat nothing but fruit), can become deficient in protein. As with most things, it is only the extremes which produce problems.

Some vegetable proteins, such as those found in soya beans and wheatgerm, are almost as good as most animal proteins. Not all animal proteins are valuable. Gelatine, for example, is so lacking in some amino acids that it could not sustain life.

The association of protein and fat was not always a problem for humans. The wild animals, seafoods and small animals which formed a major part of early human diets were rich in protein and had very little fat. The fat they did contain was largely structural fat which is polyunsaturated.

The early human diet, such as the Aboriginal diet, prior to the white's arrival in Australia, was high in protein and low in saturated fat. In Australia, shellfish, fresh and salt-water fish, crocodiles, kangaroos, lizards, goannas, turtles, wallabies, emus and other birds supplied protein, but very little fat. Contrast this with the production of fat lambs and cattle which are lot-fed to increase their weight just before slaughter. The domestication and production of obese animals has led to the contamination of protein foods with high levels of fat.

Complementary proteins

Most primitive cultures have developed eating habits which feature combinations of particular foods and these usually contain a good balance of the essential amino acids. Over a long period of time, it was probably noted that those who ate certain foods together were healthier than others. Such food combinations then became the accepted way to eat. The beans and corn eaten in Mexico, the rice and soya beans of Asia, and the couscous and chick peas of north Africa are examples of excellent food combinations where the essential amino acid missing from one food is well supplied by the other.

Many of our own food combinations also provide an excellent

balance of amino acids. Baked beans have a good protein level and
contain plenty of the amino acid lysine but lack the amino acid called
methionine. Bread happens to be a good source of methionine but is
relatively low in lysine. Together, baked beans and bread make an
excellent combination. A peanut butter sandwich or spaghetti with
cheese each combine to provide a complete set of essential amino
acids.

Good protein combinations

Cereals and legumes
> wholemeal bread with baked beans
> bread roll and pea or lentil soup
> lentil burger
> corn tacos and kidney beans
> brown rice and chick peas
> peanut butter sandwich
> rice and soya bean curd (tofu)

Cereals and dairy products
> pasta and cheese
> muesli and milk

Legumes and vegetables
> soya beans with stir–fried vegetables
> pumpkin stuffed with peas and nuts

Cereals and vegetables
> tabbouli (cracked wheat and parsley salad)
> spinach pie (wholewheat pastry base)
> vegetable or potato pies

Seeds with legumes or cereals
> lima beans with crunchy topping of sunflower seeds and
> wheatgerm
> muesli (containing pepitas or sunflower seeds and oats)

Protein powders

A variety of protein powders are available and many are marketed
specifically to athletes and those wanting to lose weight. Most consist
of either skim milk powder with added flavourings and vitamins or
protein extracted from soya beans, again with artificial flavourings
and vitamins.

These products are quite unnecessary. If used as a meal replace-
ment, many have insufficient quantities of complex carbohydrate
for anyone contemplating physical activity. Their only real use is for
hospital patients who are unable or are too weak to chew real foods
and for athletes who are too 'tied in knots' to eat a meal before an

event. Such people can sometimes manage to drink a meal when they find it difficult to swallow solid food. Since the pre–event meal will not contribute to the glycogen content of muscle, such supplements do not create problems. During training, however, they are unsuitable as meal replacements. Muscles need carbohydrate as their energy source, not protein (amino acid supplements are discussed further in chapter 12).

Food sources of protein

Foods such as fish and other seafoods, lean meat, cheese, eggs, yoghurt and milk are high in protein. Vegetable foods with a reasonably high protein content include beans of all types (baked, kidney, soya, lima and others), peas, lentils, nuts, seeds and grains. Soya bean products, such as tofu, are also high in protein. The quantities of protein in these foods are listed in Table 8.1.

How much do you need?

Estimations of the quantity of protein required by different people varies. In Western countries, the Recommended Daily Intakes (RDIs) are at the higher end of the range of levels recommended by the World Health Organization (WHO). The Western levels have been adapted to reflect usual eating patterns in these countries. The lower WHO figures would be perfectly adequate for most people.

The typical RDI for protein is one gram per kilogram of body weight. This figure takes into account variations in physical activity levels and will be adequate for even the most active people, including those involved in body building.

In general, there is no harm in eating more protein, providing that it does not come in foods which also provide fats and that total kilojoule needs are not being exceeded.

Many vegetable sources of protein have the advantage of providing complex carbohydrate in the same food as the protein. Animal protein foods have no complex carbohydrate.

A level of 10 to 15 per cent of the day's energy coming from protein is desirable. An average man should aim for a protein intake of around 75 grams a day while 60 grams will be appropriate for most women. The World Health Organization recommends a daily intake of 37 grams for men (average weight assumed to be 65 kilograms) and 29 grams for women (average weight assumed to be 55 kilograms) to meet the body's needs for good health. Appendix 1d lists the maximum amount of protein appropriate for different levels of physical activity and weight status. Check out the table of values on the following page to see how much you are eating.

91

Choose your protein

Table 8.1   Protein content of foods

Food	Protein (grams)
Meats	
Large T–bone steak, with fat	75
Lean fillet, small	35
Rump steak	60
Mince steak, 150g	30
Pork, forequarter chop, with crackling	45
loin chop, with no visible fat	21
new-fashioned, butterfly steak, no visible fat	29
Lamb, loin chop, including tail, 2	31
roast leg, no fat, average serve	44
Veal chop, 2	42
Kidneys, average serve	32
Liver, average serve	26
Sausage, grilled, 1	12
Bacon, grilled, 2 pieces	20
Ham, amount on sandwich	10
Salami, amount on sandwich	13
Meat pie or sausage roll	12
Hamburger	30
Chicken breast, average serve, no fat	34
Barbeque chicken, one quarter	24
Chicken, take-away dinner box	50
Turkey, average serve	35
Seafood	
Fish, with batter, average piece	21
grilled, average fillet	35
Oysters, 1 dozen, natural	13
Prawns, 4, king size	27
Salmon, canned, 100g	20
Tuna, canned, 100g	22
Hot potato chips, average serve	9
Dairy products	
Milk, 250mL	9
Cheese, amount on sandwich	7
Cottage cheese, half a cup	23
Icecream, regular, average serve	2
Egg, 1	6
Other	
Fruits, average piece	1
Vegetables, average serve	2
Bread, 2 slices	2
Peanuts, 25g	7
Other nuts, 25g	4

THE VEGETARIAN DIET

Pythagoras, Socrates, Plato, Aristotle, Milton, Ghandi, George Bernard Shaw, Albert Schweitzer and the gentle St Francis of Assisi were all vegetarians. Throughout the world, there are far more vegetarians than meat eaters. Most of these people are not vegetarian by choice, but have found a diet of grains, legumes, seeds, nuts, fruits and vegetables more appropriate for living conditions without refrigeration. Vegetable proteins are also cheaper than more perishable, expensive animal foods. Most of these people have perfectly adequate diets, often without many of the problems associated with our high intake of fat, salt and sugar.

Within our society, an increasing number of people are becoming vegetarian. Some believe that such a diet is healthier, others do not like the thought of killing animals for food, some have religious reasons and many are just caught up in the fashion of it all. Some sportspeople also follow a vegetarian diet so that the percentage of energy coming from complex carbohydrate will increase.

Past worries about the adequacy of a vegetarian diet usually concerned protein. With the firmly entrenched idea that protein is the most important element of the diet, many people's first concern is whether the body will suffer any deficiency without meat. The answer depends on the vegetarian foods chosen. Plants can provide every nutrient we need, including protein, provided a variety of foods is eaten.

Is it healthy?

There is no simple answer to whether a vegetarian diet is healthier than one containing meat. There is ample evidence that vegetarians have less heart disease, lower blood pressure, fewer problems with the digestive system and a lower incidence of cancer than meat eaters. However, these studies have compared vegetarians with populations who eat large quantities of animal protein foods. Comparisons with those who include only small quantities of meat or animal products may give different answers.

Just as you can have a good or bad diet which includes animal products, so there are adequate and inadequate vegetarian diets. The traditional vegetarian diet included a wide range of grains, dried beans, peas and lentils, nuts, seeds, fruits and vegetables as well as milk and eggs. It was a totally adequate and healthy way of eating.

Some 'new-style' converts to vegetarianism do not eat such a variety. Many have cut out meat in an effort to reduce their weight. Since meats are often high in kilojoules, this tactic may work.

93

However, many 'new-style' vegetarians reject healthy products such as bread, grains, nuts, cereals and legumes. Cottage cheese, lettuce and other vegetables, salads and fruits dominate the diet. These foods are fine, and should be included, but so should more concentrated foods such as grains, cereals, breads, seeds, nuts and legumes.

Nutritionists are not worried about the protein in a vegetarian diet. That is almost always adequate. They are more concerned about iron, zinc and calcium: nutrients found in plentiful supply in meat and milk. Women's iron requirements are more than double those of men (see chapter 9), so a vegetarian diet for a woman should be carefully selected to prevent iron deficiency occurring. Women are also more vulnerable to calcium losses.

The inclusion of dairy products (low fat, if desired), eggs and legumes will add important nutrients, including calcium, protein, riboflavin, iron and other minerals and vitamins. Those who omit these animal foods should ensure that they eat combinations such as those listed on page 90. For children, it is recommended that dairy products and eggs be included. If not, fortified soya milk should be a part of the diet.

Vegans

A vegetarian diet without milk, cheese, yoghurt or eggs, usually termed a vegan diet, can still meet all the body's nutritional needs. However, children and anyone with a high need for energy (such as athletes) may find it difficult to eat enough of the bulky vegetable food to provide all the nutrient needs for growth. Malnutrition is sometimes seen in vegan children, particularly if their diet is also low in fat or if there are some foods the children do not like eating.

Vitamin B_{12}, may also be in short supply if no animal products are eaten (see chapter 10). In spite of frequent medical warnings about the dangers of B_{12} deficiency, a few cases are reported regularly in children fed a vegan diet. Vitamin B_{12} has been found in mushrooms (it comes from the compost in which they are grown) and may also occur in fermented soya bean products (produced by the bacteria present in such foods) and in some drinking water. Some B_{12} may also be produced by bacteria in the intestine.

Can you eat it all?

Most vegetable foods are high in fibre, and therefore bulky. They take a long while to chew and the total quantity of food which needs to be eaten becomes large, especially for those requiring a high kilojoule intake.

Endurance athletes who train for many hours each week may

need a diet with 16 000 to 21 000 kilojoules (4000 to 5000 Calories) a day. Obtaining this quantity of food from purely low-fat vegetarian products can be difficult. It is easier if some fats from vegetable oils (preferably olive), nuts, peanuts and peanut butter are eaten along with grains, legumes, seeds, and a variety of fruits and vegetables. If possible, add some more concentrated foods such as yoghurt, cheese, milk and eggs.

A sample day of vegetarian meals

The first example of a day's vegetarian meals listed below includes dairy products and eggs. The second is for purely vegan foods. The quantities of all foods will depend on your age, size and state of physical activity.

Lacto-ovo-vegetarian menu

Breakfast
Fresh fruit or juice.
Homemade muesli or rolled oats or wholewheat breakfast biscuits with milk (low fat, if desired).
Wholemeal toast with butter, peanut butter, marmalade or honey (if desired).
Poached or boiled egg or baked beans (if desired).
Beverage (water, tea, coffee, herbal tea, milk).

Lunch
Legume or grain dish with cheese and nuts or seeds and/or pasta or potato dish.
Salad and/or cooked vegetables.
Wholemeal bread with butter, margarine or avocado.
Fruit.

Evening meal
Similar selection to lunch but with variations to include wide range of foods.

Snacks
Milk, cheese, breads, wholegrain crispbread, fresh or dried fruits, nuts or seeds.

Drinks
Water, fruit juices, milk.

Vegan menu

Breakfast
Porridge made with soya milk and honey or homemade muesli served with fruit and juice.

95

Wholemeal toast with margarine or peanut butter, honey or jam (if
  desired).
Baked beans or sweet corn or tomatoes and mushrooms.
Beverage (water, tea, coffee, herbal tea, soya milk).

Lunch
Legume or grain dish with nuts or seeds and/or pasta or potato dish.
Salad and/or cooked vegetables.
Wholemeal bread with margarine or avocado.
Fruit.

Evening meal
Similar selection to lunch, but with the type of dish varied so that a
  wide selection of legumes, grains, nuts and seeds are included.

Snacks
Soya milk, breads, wholegrain crispbread, fresh or dried fruits, nuts
  or seeds.

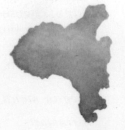

9

Iron, calcium and other minerals

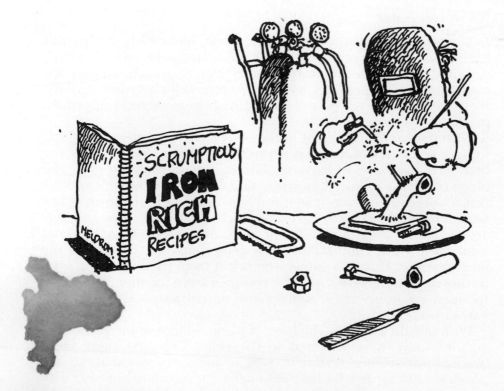

MANY people take vitamin supplements in their quest for an antidote to a poor diet. In spite of the proliferation of junk foods, few people suffer from vitamin deficiencies. A lack of particular minerals in the daily diet gives much greater cause for concern.

Minerals are important constituents of the blood: they take part in various chemical reactions, strengthen the bones and are involved in the functioning of nerves and muscles. All the minerals needed are available from foods, provided the right foods are chosen.

IRON

Only relatively small amounts of iron, the equivalent of a large nail, are stored in the body. But that tiny four grams of iron is vital for good health and peak performance. A lack of iron is the most common nutritional deficiency in the world. It is not confined to third-world countries, but occurs in a significant number of women in developed countries. Female athletes need to pay particular attention to their iron supplies.

What does it do?

Iron has many functions in the body. In red blood cells, it is part of haemoglobin which carries oxygen to all body tissues and takes back carbon dioxide to the lungs. In muscles, iron is an essential part of a compound which provides oxygen for strenuous physical activity. Iron is also an essential part of the chain of chemical reactions which produce energy in the body.

With such an involvement in the body's energy systems, it's little wonder that a lack of iron makes you tired. About 75 per cent of the body's iron is found in haemoglobin, the pigment which gives red blood cells their colour. A small amount of iron is in the cells and the rest is stored in the liver, spleen and bone marrow in the form of ferritin. The red blood cells have a life cycle of 120 days and each day around 2000 million red blood cells die. Their iron becomes available for the 2000 million new cells which are formed in the bone marrow. However, some iron is lost from the skin and the intestine each day and this must be replaced from the diet. The losses for men are quite small; women lose much more. Aspirin causes extra iron losses.

With insufficient iron, the level of haemoglobin in the blood falls and less oxygen is delivered to the cells. The first signs are a 'washed-out' feeling, weakness, fatigue and a decreased ability for physical acitivity. A full-blown iron deficiency leads to anaemia with symptoms of weakenss, shortness of breath, coldness, palpitations and 'pins and needles' in the feet. In extreme cases, anaemia can cause difficulty in swallowing and even death.

A measurement of the haemoglobin in the blood shows whether anaemia is a problem. Measuring the ferritin stores is also important as these closely reflect the amount of available iron in a person's diet. Women generally have lower ferritin levels than men. Those who have had a number of pregnancies tend to have the lowest iron stores.

A recent report has linked iron deficiency in children with restlessness, inability to concentrate and irritability. Treatment with iron rapidly reversed these problems.

Women and iron

A lack of iron is common in women, including women athletes. It is much rarer in men. This apparent sexist bias arises because women need more than twice as much iron as men due to loss of blood (and hence iron) during menstruation. Pregnancy and lactation impose even greater losses. During a period, a woman loses about as much iron as is normally lost in a month. Pregnancy means nine period-free months, but the loss of iron to the baby is equivalent to the amount normally lost in almost twice as many menstrual periods.

In spite of their much greater need for iron, women have traditionally taken the smallest share of the best food source of iron : lean meat. We have campaigns to 'Feed the Man Meat' and even small boys are encouraged to eat more meat than their sisters. Women need the iron; men eat the meat. Why not 'Feed the Woman Meat'!

Many women who feel chronically tired and somewhat irritable should check whether they have a mild lack of iron. Even though iron deficiency is the most common health problem in the world, it is often misdiagnosed as 'a woman's lot' or ignored because the symptoms seem too vague.

Chronic tiredness *may* be due to a lack of sleep or a basic unhappiness with life. But it could be due to a lack of iron. A woman who constantly feels 'worn out', has heavy menstrual periods, or has an intra–uterine device fitted, or has had several pregnancies should ask her doctor to check for iron deficiency.

From recent surveys, it has been estimated that many women eat less than 10 milligrams of iron a day. Many teenage girls have an ever lower intake. Such low quantities of iron can lead to iron deficiency.

Special problems for slimmers

Many women are so obsessed with achieving extreme slenderness that they eat very little. This new ultra-thin image is responsible for the iron content of the average woman's diet falling to a new low

99

level. The result may be a slim body with frequent fatigue due to low iron stores.

It is almost impossible for any very strict diet to supply enough iron. Even those who are simply health conscious can go to extremes. Discovering the high kilojoule content of a T-bone steak, many women opt for a totally meatless diet. This would be fine if a range of legumes, grains, breads and vegetables are consumed. But in many cases, the health-conscious woman will simply skip all meat and eat nothing in its place.

It makes far better sense to eat small portions of very lean meats. As you can see from the table of iron values on page 103, it is possible to take in sufficient iron without eating meat, but it is more difficult.

Here are two examples of typical meals eaten by health-conscious women and their approximate iron contents. Note that even foods which are healthy in other respects may not contain sufficient iron.

Menu 1

Breakfast: Glass of fresh orange juice
Bowl of fresh fruit
Lunch: Salad
Piece of cheese
Carton of yoghurt
Piece of fruit
Dinner: Stir-fried vegetables

This menu contains less than six milligrams : far too little for good health.

Menu 2

Breakfast: Bowl of cereal with milk
Slice of wholemeal toast
Piece of fresh fruit
Lunch: Large salad
Wholemeal roll
Apple
Dinner: 150g of grilled fish
Potato and two steamed vegetables
Fresh fruit salad

This menu has approximately thirteen milligrams of iron, and just scrapes into the recommended daily intake.

How much do you need?

Requirements for iron are increased if blood is lost, or when more blood is required, as occurs during growth. Menstruation doubles a woman's iron requirements compared with a man's while pregnancy and childbirth make even greater demands. Children's needs are high to meet the demands of growth.

The recommended daily intakes of iron are as follows:

	Age or stage of life	Milligrams of iron
Women	18–54	12
	54+	7
	During pregnancy	13
	During lactation	15
Men		10
Boys	1–11	7–10
	12–18	12
Girls	1–11	6–8
	12–18	10–13

Can you have too much iron?

As with most nutrients, it is possible to take in too much iron, but it is very rare and likely to occur from taking an overdose of iron pills. Much of this exces is not absorbed but causes gastrointestinal problems and diarrhoea.

Zinc and iron can interact in the human diet. Too much iron can reduce the amount of zinc which can be absorbed. This has been found with people taking supplements of more than 30 milligrams of iron a day. Some commonly sold supplements contain many times more iron than zinc and can lead to a zinc deficiency.

The Bantu tribes in Africa suffer from iron overload caused by brewing potent beer in iron pots. The alcohol causes the pots to dissolve and the Bantu people experience a severe disease called haemochromatosis, in which the liver and pancreas cease to function properly.

Types of iron

Foods contain iron in two main forms. Meat, seafoods, and poultry have haem iron. Cereals, vegetables and eggs contain non-haem iron. The haem iron is absorbed much better than the non-haem variety. Most women will find it easier to meet their iron requirements if they include some meat, seafoods or poultry.

The absorption of iron

The non-haem iron is absorbed to a much greater extent if some haem iron is present at the same meal or if a food containing vitamin C is eaten at the same meal. For example, if you have a poached egg on a slice of wholemeal toast, you will not absorb much of the iron from either food. However, if you add some type of fruit or vegetable (perhaps a glass of orange juice, a slice of melon or some tomato), the iron in the egg and toast will be more useful to your body. For this reason alone, it makes good sense to include a fruit or vegetable at each meal so that the vitamin C present will assist the body to absorb iron from other foods.

The amount of iron absorbed depends on how much is needed. If you lack iron, the body cleverly absorbs more. During pregnancy, when needs are especially high, iron absorption can almost double. Children who are finicky eaters and appear to eat very little also absorb much more iron from foods.

Other factors in foods also influence iron absorption. Cereal grains contain a substance called phytic acid which 'ties up' minerals such as iron, making them unavailable to the body. Most wholegrain cereals are so much richer in iron than their processed counterparts that, even accounting for the effect of the phytic acid present, they still contribute iron to the diet. Wholemeal and wholegrain breads do not present any problems. The yeast used in making bread prevents the phytic acid from forming complexes with minerals. Problems can arise, however, with foods which may contribute so much phytic acid that iron deficiency becomes one of a number of possible problems. It is wise not to eat more than one to two level tablespoons of unprocessed bran a day.

Other substances present in foods can also 'tie up' iron so that it is not absorbed. Oxalic acid in spinach, for example, makes the Popeye story a bit of a myth since not much of the iron in spinach escapes the clutches of the oxalic acid. Popeye's great strength certainly did not come from spinach.

The tannin in well-brewed tea can also interfere with iron absorption. Unless you like your tea fairly weak and poured quickly from the pot after it is made, it is best to confine tea drinking to between meals.

Where do you find iron?

Iron occurs in oysters, red meats (especially liver and kidneys), poultry, fish, egg yolk, green leafy vegetables, cereals and wholemeal bread, dried fruits, legumes and nuts. Anyone who cooks in iron pots will also get iron from the pot. Vegetarians *can* obtain sufficient iron if they eat a variety of legumes, grains, seeds, nuts and vegetables.

Check your daily iron intake, using the following values:

Table 9.1   Food sources of iron

Food	Iron content (milligrams)
Liver, 100g	8.8
Kidney, 100g	9.2
Liverwurst, 40g	2.1
Steak, lean, 150g	4.5
Lamb, loin chops, 2, average	2.0
Pork, steak, average size	1.2
Veal, steak, 150g	2.7
Chicken or turkey, 150g	1.4
Fish, average fillet, 150g	2.1
Salmon, canned, 100g	1.4
Oysters, 1 dozen	7.2
Wholemeal bread, 1 slice	1.0
White bread, 1 slice	0.4
Breakfast cereal, average serve	2.5
Rolled oats, average serve	1.8
Wheatgerm, 1 tablespoon	0.8
Egg, 1	1.1
Cheese, 30g	0.2
Milk, regular or low fat, 1 cup	0.2
Yoghurt, natural or fruit, small carton	0.2
Lentils, dried beans, cooked, half a cup	1.8
Broccoli, 100g, steamed	1.0
Peas, fresh, frozen or canned, half a cup	1.1
Carrot, 1, small	0.6
Vegetables, average serve	0.8
Salad vegetables, average plate	1.2
Potato, 1, medium	0.8
Fruit, average piece	0.5
Orange juice, 200mL	0.6
Dried apricots, 50g	2.0

Iron supplements

It is usually best to obtain nutrients from food. However, if you lack iron, supplements can correct the deficiency.

Women who have heavy periods may need an iron supplement. Have your haemoglobin and ferritin levels checked to find out if a supplement is needed.

Look for a supplement which contains vitamin C as this will help the iron to be absorbed or take an iron supplement with meals so that the vitamin C from fruits and vegetables can assist absorption of the iron from the supplement.

Some iron supplements contain too little iron to be useful. Many people also find that iron tablets upset their digestive system and cause either diarrhoea or constipation. If this is the case, try a 103

different supplement until you find one which suits your body. Take
only the recommended dose.

For peak performance

- Eat some lean meat (about 100 grams cooked weight) a day or choose
some good vegetarian alternatives.
- Include a range of foods such as wholemeal bread, green leafy
vegetables, eggs and dried fruits.
- If you suspect iron deficiency, have a doctor check your haemoglobin
and ferritin levels.

CALCIUM: THE BONE MINERAL

Calcium has made a comeback. Years ago, people used to encourage
children to drink milk so that their bones would grow strong. Once
past childhood, however, calcium was largely ignored. It was
assumed that when bones had finished growing, calcium was of little
importance.

How wrong such ideas were. Current studies of the density and
strength of women's bones have shown that calcium is vitally
important throughout life. All parts of the body are in a constant
state of turnover, and that includes the bones. The minerals which
give bones their hardness are constantly moving in and out of the
skeleton.

Why do we need it?

Calcium is not only needed by the bones: a certain level must be
present in the blood for the nerves and muscles to function
properly. The blood calcium has narrow limits and cannot vary
much. If it drops even a little, the body will withdraw some of the
calcium from the bones to make up the correct concentration of
calcium in the blood. As far as the body is concerned, the bones are a
reservoir of calcium.

If insufficient calcium is absorbed into the bones, it is easy for the
losses of calcium to be a little greater than the intake. The result is a
slow but steady loss of bone calcium. After a number of years, the
bones become less dense, lose some of their strength and the
condition known as osteoporosis, or porous bones, occurs.

Special problems of women

Both men and women tend to lose calcium from their skeletons as
they age. Women, however, suffer about twice the calcium loss that
is experienced by men. This makes osteoporosis and bone fractures
common in older women.

Around the menopause, changes in female hormones accelerate the loss of calcium from the bones. The denser the bones are to start with, the less the likelihood of enough calcium being lost to cause osteoporosis. It is therefore important for women to have built up sufficient calcium in the skeleton over the previous 20 to 30 years.

There are not many good things which can be said about excess weight. However, it does offer protection against weak bones, while the fashion for extreme thinness in women increases the risk. Those women who either eat so little or exercise so much that their body fat levels drop so low that they stop menstruating have a double problem. They do not build up the strong skeleton which is needed for later life, and they begin to suffer the withdrawal of calcium which normally does not occur until menopause. This problem occurs in very thin women and also in elite women athletes. It can be avoided by keeping body fat levels high enough for normal menstrual periods to occur.

The retention of calcium

Large quantities of calcium are found only in a few foods. To make it even more difficult, there are a number of factors which interfere with the retention of this valuable mineral. Some of the factors which influence calcium retention are:

The amount of calcium in the diet: Sounds obvious, but you cannot absorb calcium unless you are taking it into the body. See the table on pages 108–109 for food sources of calcium.

Vitamin D: This vitamin is essential for calcium to be used by the body. In some countries where the winter is so long and cold that the skin is not exposed to the sun, vitamin D must be obtained from butter, margarine or fish liver oils. It is well supplied in sunny countries and deficiencies rarely occur.

Phosphorus: This mineral is also essential for strong bones. Too much phosphorus, however, can increase the loss of calcium from bones. It would be foolish to take phosphorus supplements as almost all our foods supply it.

Hormones: At different ages, a deficiency of female hormones has two major effects on bones. During adolescence and the early adult years, a decrease in hormone levels means that the bones do not accumulate as much calcium. Around menopause, the normal decrease in hormone levels increases the amount of calcium withdrawn from the bones.

Exercise: Weight-bearing exercise is vital for calcium to be absorbed into the bones. Our modern lifestyle discourages weight-bearing activity. Most of us drive instead of walking. Few of us do any heavy

105

housework, our work activities tend to involve sitting or standing, and our leisure activities rarely involve strenuous physical activity. Walking, carrying groceries or other items, dancing, running, walking up stairs, aerobics, skipping or active sports will increase calcium absorption. Swimming is generally thought to have less benefits for bones. However, recent evidence suggests that some types of swimming, especially backstroke, exert a pull on the bones in the spine which will encourage calcium to be deposited.

Protein: A high protein intake means that less calcium is absorbed. Doubling the protein from 50 to 100 grams a day will almost halve the amount of calcium absorbed. For this reason, very large serves of meat or other high-protein foods are inadvisable. A well-balanced diet should contain enough protein, but not excessive quantities.

Salt: A high salt intake also accelerates calcium loss. So, go easy with the salt: there is plenty present naturally in foods and you do not need to add any.

Caffeine: Drinking lots of coffee can interfere with calcium absorption. Caffeine also occurs in cola drinks, tea and chocolate.

Oxalic acid: Found in sesame seeds, spinach and rhubarb, both oxalic acid and the phytic acid in cereals can 'tie up' calcium so that it cannot be absorbed. Both spinach and rhubarb have a high content of calcium and even though their oxalic acid will 'tie up' some of this calcium, they are unlikely to affect the calcium in other foods eaten at the same meal. Celery leaves are also high in oxalic acid and it is not advisable to eat large quantities of them.

Nicotine and alcohol: These drugs also reduce calcium absorption. Keep alcohol intake to a minimum and avoid smoking altogether.

How much calcium do you need?

	Age or stage of life	Recommended calcium intake (milligrams)
Women		500
	After menopause	500
	During pregnancy	1200
	During lactation	1200
Men		500
Infants	Up to 6 months	600
Children	1–7 years	600
Girls	8–11 years	700
	12–15 years	700
	16–18 years	500
Boys	8–11 years	600
	12–15 years	700
	16–18 years	600

Where is calcium found?

Calcium is in milk, cheese and yoghurt. Smaller quantities are found in green vegetables, seafoods, nuts, oranges and soya beans.

The most convenient source of calcium is some type of milk, cheese or yoghurt (either from cows, sheep, goats or buffalo). In many countries, much of the calcium comes from eating small fish which are dried or minced up, bones and all, and used in a soup. This provides an excellent source of calcium. In other areas, soya beans are the major source.

Humans are the only mammals who continue to drink milk after they are weaned. This is because humans are the only animals who continue to produce the enzyme to digest lactose or milk sugar. This adaptation is thought to have occurred over several thousand years in populations who have continued to drink milk. In some parts of the world where milk is not used, most people stop producing this enzyme and are unable to digest milk. These groups include many Asian people, some Australian Aborigines and Pacific Island groups and people from Middle Eastern countries and southern Europe.

Each of these groups has some other source of dietary calcium. Asians rely on soya beans and fish, Australian Aborigines used various seafoods and obtained some calcium from plants, seeds and nuts, while people from many other areas used sheep's or goat's milk to produce cheeses (which have little lactose).

What happens if you don't like milk?

It is easy to take in sufficient calcium by drinking milk and the combination of calcium and lactose present helps calcium to be absorbed. Low-fat milks contain just as much (and sometimes more) calcium as regular milk. Cooking with milk does not destroy its calcium.

If you do not like milk or if you have an allergy or a sensitivity to it, you can use green leafy vegetables, oranges, fish (especially canned or dried fish with edible bones) and almonds to supply calcium. A supplement may be necessary for those with high calcium requirements.

Cheese can supply calcium, and many people who need to avoid milk because of its lactose will be able to eat cheese. The only cheese with significant quantities of lactose is ricotta. Yoghurt is also a valuable source of calcium.

Some people maintain that sesame seeds are an excellent source of calcium. So they are, but only if you eat them complete with husks! The usual sesame seeds we buy have had their husks removed (they are 'decorticated'). To obtain sufficient calcium from decorticated sesame seeds you would need to eat about 50 teaspoons a day! That's a lot of munching, and a heap of fat would accompany the calcium.

107

When is it too late to start considering calcium?

There is some dispute about whether calcium is absorbed by women after the menopause. Some studies indicate that calcium can still be absorbed into bones; others maintain that an oestrogen supplement is necessary for older women to absorb enough calcium to strengthen bones. Nutritionists recommend that people of all ages have an adequate calcium intake.

Calcium supplements

Calcium supplements contain varying quantities of calcium. In general, their calcium is not absorbed as well as that in milk. However, they can be useful for people who cannot drink milk.

What about excess calcium?

It is unlikely that too much calcium will come from food. Exceeding the recommended dose of a supplement can supply too much calcium. Normally any excess calcium will not be absorbed by the body. In some people, however, the hormones which control the absorption of calcium may not function properly and too much calcium can cause kidney stones.

Where can you find calcium?

Table 9.2   Calcium content of foods

Food	Amount of calcium (milligrams)
Milk (including skim) 250mL	290
Shape or low fat milk, 250mL	400
Yoghurt, 200g, natural	380
Weight Watchers, natural	480
fruit	305
Weight Watchers, fruit	350
Cheese, 30g	260
Cottage cheese, 100g	75
Almonds, 50g	125
Sesame seed kernels, 10g	15
Sesame seeds, with hulls, 20g	200
Sesame paste (tahini), made from whole sesame seeds, 20g	190
Sesame paste, made from sesame kernel, 20g	85
Salmon, 100g	185
Tuna, 100g	10
Fresh fish fillet, 150g	90
Oysters, 6	145
Soya beans, cooked, 1 cup	130

Table 9.2 Calcium content of foods — continued

Food	Amount of calcium (milligrams)
Soya bean milk, 1 cup	55
So good, 1 cup	290
Soya bean curd (tofu), 100g	130
Egg, 1	35
Orange, medium, 1	50
Fruit, average piece	10
Broccoli, 100g	125
Cabbage, 100g	50
Most vegetables, average serve	35
Baked beans, 50g	20
Most breakfast cereals, 20g	15
Bread, 1 slice	10

Hints for increasing calcium

1 Use low fat milk on your breakfast cereal.
2 Include a salmon sandwich and a glass of low-fat milk often at lunch.
3 Make a frothy low-fat milkshake by blending a glass of skim milk, a couple of icecubes, some vanilla and/or a banana.
4 Have a glass of low-fat milk (hot or cold) in place of a cup of tea or coffee at night.
5 Add skim milk powder to vegetable soups to produce a thick creamy texture.
6 Use yoghurt in place of sour cream on potatoes and fruit: it saves fat and adds calcium.
7 If you do not like skim milk, it could be because you are using a powdered product. Try fresh skim milk or brands of low fat milk.

For peak performance

- Include some weight-bearing exercise in your daily routine.
- Make sure you take in your daily needs of calcium.
- For women: to prevent calcium loss from bones, do not allow body fat levels to go so low that your periods cease.

ZINC

Many people think of zinc as the stuff that stops the roof rusting and keeps your nose from getting sunburnt at the beach. About 25 years ago, zinc was recognised as an essential nutrient for humans. It cannot be made in the human body but must be supplied from the diet. The body contains two to three grams of zinc, with the greatest amounts being found in the liver, kidney, brain and pancreas.

What does it do?

Like most minerals, zinc is a vital part of many of the enzymes which control various chemical reactions in the body. It is important for wound healing, essential for growth and normal sexual development, helps the body to make protein and to use carbohydrates efficiently and keeps the membranes around cells in a healthy condition. This does not mean that a person taking extra zinc will grow taller, have perfect skin or super sexual prowess: these are all common claims made by some promoters of zinc supplements.

A deficiency of zinc is not uncommon, even in Western countries. Its symptoms include a loss of taste sensation, slow healing of injuries to the skin, failure to grow normally (in children) and a decreased sperm count.

Since alcohol causes a lot of zinc to be lost in the urine, heavy drinkers can develop zinc deficiency. This problem is not confined to skid-row alcoholics; it can occur in those who have a good diet, but drink a lot of alcohol.

A lack of zinc can be diagnosed by determining the levels of zinc in certain types of blood cells. Hair analysis is *not* a reliable test and commonly used tests measuring the amount of zinc in blood plasma do not give a true indication of zinc deficiency.

How much do you need?

Too much zinc, as with all minerals, can be as harmful as too little. Requirements for zinc increase during growth, pregnancy and lactation. In Australia the Recommended Daily Intake is as follows:

	Age or stage of life	Milligrams of zinc
Infants		3–6
Children	1–3 years	4.5–6
	4–7 years	6–9
	8–11 years	9–14
	12–18 years	12–18
Adults		12–16
	During pregnancy	16–21
	During lactation	18–24

In Britain, deficiency of zinc is rare and the Department of Health and Social Security have not set recommended amounts.

The Recommended Daily Intakes of zinc assume that the diet contains both animal and vegetable foods. Strict vegetarians will need to eat a little more total zinc since some of the zinc in their vegetable foods is poorly absorbed.

Zinc is lost in sweat and athletes engaged in strenuous physical training should aim for the upper level of zinc.

Can you have too much zinc?

Zinc is potentially a toxic mineral and excess can come from industrial contamination or from over-zealous use of zinc supplements. These can also have a secondary effect of causing iron deficiency and interfering with the body's ability to use other minerals, such as copper.

Symptoms of zinc excess include dehydration, diarrhoea, nausea, abdominal pains, dizziness, a lack of muscular coordination and feelings of lethargy.

It is most unlikely that anyone would have an overdose of zinc from foods, but mega-dose supplements are hazardous. A dose equal to 10 times the daily needs is dangerous.

The absorption of zinc

Like other minerals, the amount of zinc absorbed depends on several factors. To some extent, the more zinc you need, the more you can absorb. Anyone who has been fasting will absorb large quantities: a potential danger for those who fast and take supplements.

Phytic acid and phosphates present in soya beans and wholegrain cereal products can interfere with zinc absorption. Those who use soya products in preference to foods such as milk and meat will absorb less zinc. This can be a problem in children. Taking large quantities of unprocessed bran can also lead to zinc deficiency. One to two tablespoons of bran a day is fine; larger quantities should be avoided.

A factor in breast milk also increases the amount of zinc which is absorbed. Cow's milk has much more zinc than human milk, yet breastfed babies absorb more.

Where do you find zinc?

Cassanova is reputed to have had a permanent love affair with oysters. Noting the amount of zinc in these delectable bivalves shows that he certainly would not have suffered zinc deficiency!

In general, the zinc in animal foods is absorbed better than that in vegetable sources.

111

Zinc content of foods

Table 9.3 Food sources of zinc

Food	Zinc (milligrams)
Oysters, 6	27.0
Mussels, 6	1.9
Fish, 150g	1.5
Sardines, 100g	3.0
Steak, 150g	6.9
Sausages, average, 2	2.4
Chicken, breast, 100g	0.8
leg, 100g	2.4
Veal, steak, 150g	4.8
Pork, steak, average size	2.2
Lamb chops, average, 2	2.6
Egg, 1	1.0
Cheese, 30g	1.2
Cottage cheese, 100g	0.5
Milk, regular or skim, 250mL	1.0
Rolled oats, average serve	2.3
Bread, wholemeal, 2 slices	1.0
white, 2 slices	0.4
Breakfast cereal, average bowl	0.8
Bran, 10g	1.6
Baked beans, 200g	1.4
Broccoli, 100g	0.5
Carrot, medium, 1	0.6
Lentils, 100g uncooked weight	3.0
Peas, 75g	0.5
Potato, medium, 1	0.4
Other vegetables, average serve	0.2
Fruit, average piece	0.2
Brazil nuts, 50g	2.1
Hazelnuts, 50g	1.2
Peanuts, 50g	1.5
Peanut butter, 25g	0.8
Walnuts, 50g	1.5

For peak performance

- Make sure that your diet has sufficient zinc, but avoid excessive quantities in supplements.
- Try to have a mixture of both animal and vegetable foods so that more zinc will be absorbed.
- Avoid taking more than one to two tablespoons of unprocessed bran a day.

POTASSIUM

This mineral is important to balance the sodium obtained from salt. Potassium is richly supplied by fruits and vegetables, but is low in most highly processed foods. The average body contains 100 to 140 grams of potassium, the amount decreasing with age and increasing body fat levels. The mineral is concentrated in the lean tissue of the body and trained athletes have greater quantities.

What does it do?

Potassium is found inside body cells while sodium is mainly outside the body cells in the plasma of the blood and in the spaces between cells. The distribution of sodium and potassium is controlled by the kidney and regulates the amount of water inside and around the cells. Too much sodium (from salt) draws water out of the cells, raising the concentration of potassium within the cells. It is thought that eating foods with a higher potassium content will prevent this imbalance.

Potassium is also important in the transmission of nerve impulses, including those which cause muscle cells to contract. The heart muscle is affected by a lack of potassium.

A dietary lack of potassium is rare. Deficiency usually occurs after prolonged diarrhoea or vomiting (for example, in those with eating disorders such as anorexia or binge eating) or when the kidneys are not functioning properly. Diuretics, laxatives and fasting also cause a loss of potassium.

Athletes need to ensure that their diet contains plenty of potassium. Extra losses of the mineral can occur with heavy and prolonged sweating and a lack will cause muscle weakness, fatigue and abnormal heart rhythms.

How much do you need?

Potassium is easily obtained from foods. Supplements should only be used in conjunction with some diuretics. In Australia, Recommended Daily Intakes are as follows, but recommended amounts have not been set in Britain:

	Age or Stage of life	Millimoles of potassium
Infants	Up to 6 months	10–15 (400–600mg)
	7–12 months	12–35 (480–1400mg)
Children	1–3 years	25–70 (1000–2800mg)
	4–7 years	40–100 (1600–4000mg)
	8–18 years	50–140 (2000–5600mg)
Adults		50–140 (2000–5600mg)
	65+ years	40–130 (1600–5200mg)
	During pregnancy	50–140 (2000–5600mg)
	During lactation	65–140 (2600–5600mg)

113

Where do you find potassium?

Potassium is found in meats, vegetables and fruits, milk, legumes and cereals. By eating several kinds of vegetables a day, two to three pieces of fruit, and a variety of other foods, you will obtain plenty of potassium.

If the diet consists of highly processed foods, the amount of potassium may be insufficient. Nature provides foods with a little sodium and plenty of potassium; food manufacturers remove much of the potassium and add large quantities of sodium. This destroys the natural balance.

If you wish to check out the potassium in your diet, the following figures will help.

Table 9.4   Food sources of potassium

Food	Potassium (milligrams)
Steak, lean, 150g	750
Chicken, 150g	415
Lamb chops, average, 2	260
Fish, average fillet	580
Egg, 1	85
Milk, regular or low fat, 250mL	375
Cheese, 30g	40
Bread, wholemeal, 2 slices	110
white, 2 slices	50
Unprocessed bran, 10g	120
Wheatgerm, 10g	100
Cereal, average bowl, high-fibre type	200
highly processed	30
Rice, average serve	90
Spaghetti, average serve	140
Baked beans, 200g	600
Chick peas, 100g raw weight	800
Mushrooms, 100g	470
Parsley, 100g	1080
Potato, 1, medium, steamed	450
1, large, baked in jacket	990
Raw vegetables, 100g, average	350
Cooked vegetables, 100g, average	220
Apple, medium	170
Banana, medium	380
Orange, medium	270
Rhubarb, average serve, stewed	540
Tomato juice, 250ml	650
Average for most fresh fruits	250
Dried fruits, 50g, average	450
Prunes, 50g	700
Nuts, 50g	400
Cocoa powder, 10g	150

For peak performance

- Eat plenty of fruit and vegetables (including some raw) to provide potassium.

- Keep salt intake low to preserve the balance of potassium inside the cells.

- Avoid sports drinks which contain too much potassium: the maximum concentration should be 100 milligrams per litre.

MAGNESIUM

Much of the body's 25 milligrams of magnesium occurs in the bones. Some is also inside the body cells where it takes part in the chemical reactions involved in the release of energy.

Why do we need it?

Like many other minerals, magnesium is involved in the enzyme systems which control the way the body uses proteins, fats and carbohydrates. It is also important in nerves and muscles and contributes hardness and rigidity to bones.

Magnesium deficiency is rare in humans partly because the mineral is widely distributed in foods and partly because the kidneys have a highly efficient system for conserving it. However, diarrhoea and vomiting may cause severe losses.

The most common cause of magnesium deficiency occurs in those who drink a lot of alcohol. Symptoms include loss of appetite, nausea, tremor, excessive irritability of nerves and muscles, and seizures.

This latter symptom has led some people to advise epileptics to take large doses of magnesium to control their symptoms. There is no sound medical evidence that this is effective.

There has also been a claim that taking magnesium is valuable for heart problems. People with high blood pressure have lower levels of magesium in the body and there is much less heart disease in areas where the water is hard and has a high content of magesium. It has also been shown that extra magnesium is valuable after open heart surgery.

The conclusion of reputable medical researchers is that magnesium has an important role in keeping the heart healthy. However, problems due to a lack of magnesium are usually secondary to a high alcohol consumption or a consequence of taking diuretics rather than due to a dietary lack.

115

How much do you need?

The following figures represent the Recommended Daily Intakes of magnesium for Australians but recommended amounts have not been set in Britain.

	Age or stage of life	Milligrams of magnesium
Infants	0–6 months	40
	7–12 months	60
Children	1–3 years	80
	4–7 years	110
Boys	8–11 years	180
	12–15 years	260
	16+	320
Girls	8–11 years	160
	12–15 years	240
	16+	270
Men		320
Women		270
	During pregnancy	300
	During lactation	340

Can you have too much magnesium?

As long as the kidneys are functioning, it is unlikely that too much magnesium from food sources would be harmful. Very high doses (which may come from antacids and laxatives) can lead to very low blood pressure, weakness and depression.

Where is it found?

Magnesium occurs in cereals, meats, dairy products, fruits and vegetables. If you wish to check on your daily intake, the major food sources are listed below.

Table 9.5 Magnesium content of foods

Food	Magnesium (milligrams)
Unprocessed bran, 10g	50
Wheatgerm, 10g	20
Bran cereal, average serve	220
Breakfast cereal, high-fibre type	60
highly processed	5
Rolled oats, average serve	70
Bread, wholemeal, 2 slices	45
white, 2 slices	15
Spaghetti, average serve	35

Table 9.5　Magnesium content of foods — continued

Food	Magnesium (milligrams)
Milk, regular or low fat, 250mL	40
Chicken, average, 150g	35
Steak, 150g	30
Lamb chops, average, 2	20
Fish, average fillet, 150g	45
Sardines, 100g	50
Dried beans or peas, 100g raw weight	180
Baked beans, canned, 200g	60
Corn, medium cob	50
Spinach, cooked, 100g	60
Vegetables, cooked, 100g average	15
raw, 100g average	10
Banana, medium	55
Most fresh fruits, average piece	10
Dried fruit, 50g	30
Berry fruits, half a punnet	40

10

Vitamins:
Food or pills?

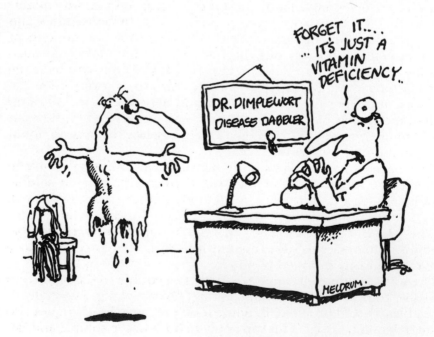

PEOPLE in Western countries tend to be great pill-poppers and many men (and often even more women) now like to take vitamin supplements. To many people, nutrition means taking vitamins.

There are few cases of frank vitamin deficiencies in most Western countries and the variety of foods available can easily contribute all the vitamins the body needs. So why is so much money spent on vitamin pills?

Most people take vitamin pills for nutritional insurance. If you do not know which foods contain vitamins and if you believe the vitamin manufacturers who maintain that today's foods are deficient in these vital nutrients, a bottle of pills seems the easiest course of action. A recent survey found that more than half of the population has been conned by this nutritional insurance theory.

There is also a popular belief that vitamins will provide extra energy and perk you up when you feel down. One study found that only 12 per cent of adults were aware that vitamins do *not* provide the body with a direct source of energy.

What do vitamins do?

Vitamins are essential organic substances required in minute quantities so that we can process the proteins, fats, carbohydrates and minerals from the foods that we eat. They are vital components of the enzymes which carry out the body's basic functions and most must be obtained from the foods that we eat (a couple can be made by bacteria in the intestine). Without vitamins, various chemical reactions in the body will not proceed and deficiencies will show up in malfunctioning blood cells, disorders of the skin, eyes, nervous and immune systems. With so many roles to play, there is no doubt that vitamins are important.

There are two major classes of vitamins: those which dissolve in fat and those which are soluble in water. In general, the fat-soluble vitamins (A, D, E and K) stay in the body (either in the liver or in body fat) for much longer than those vitamins which are water soluble (the B–complex and C). A regular supply of water-soluble vitamins is thus essential. Fortunately, this creates no problems since they can be easily supplied by foods.

The water-soluble vitamins are more susceptible to damage from excessive heat or water used in cooking. Overcooking, especially of vegetables, should be avoided. Some food processing techniques also result in vitamin losses. This can apply to both water-soluble and fat-soluble vitamins. The water-soluble are primarily lost by heat while some of the fat-soluble vitamins are lost when various parts of foods are removed during processing. Turning wheat grains into white flour, for example, means that most of the vitamin E is lost.

119

However, if other food sources of vitamin E are consumed, for example wheatgerm, this loss can be accommodated. In general, whole foods have a better retention of vitamins, at least until they enter the home kitchen. In spite of the protestations of those implacably opposed to food processing, more vitamin loss probably occurs in the home kitchen than in many food processing methods.

It has been known for years that the fat-soluble vitamins are potentially dangerous if taken in large doses since the body's safe storage sites are limited. However, we now know that even though excess quantities of water-soluble vitamins can be excreted in the urine, mega-doses of these can damage the body before they are passed out.

The vitamin content of various foods differs, depending on the time of growth, harvesting, storage and processing methods. There is also some individual variation between, say, one carrot and another. The same situation exists with the protein, fat, carbohydrate and water content of various foods. This natural variation is not a reason to take your vitamins from a pill rather than from foods. Foods do not produce vitamins just for our benefit: vitamins are vital to their own structures and functions. If a plant does not receive the nutrients it needs, it simply does not grow. So, produce which reaches maturity does not lack vitamins even though any one plant may have a little more or a little less of a particular vitamin than its neighbour. These perfectly natural variations are taken into account when foods are analysed for their vitamin content.

Supplements: miracle or menace?

Cars will not go without petrol, but a car will not go any better if you try to pour more petrol into the tank than it will hold. In fact, the petrol spilling over the car's body and paintwork can cause problems. Vitamins are similar. You need enough for the body to function properly, but taking excess amounts will not make your body work any better. And just as extra petrol will not make up for a lack of oil in your car's engine, neither will taking extra vitamins make up for neglect in other areas of your daily diet. Vitamin deficiencies are rare in Western countries. In fact, the excess consumption of vitamins is probably a greater problem than any deficiency.

There are occasions where supplementary vitamins can be useful. In general, though, any diet which lacks vitamins is almost certainly unbalanced. Contrary to popular belief and much of the advertising by vitamin manufacturers, you cannot correct an unbalanced diet with vitamin pills. Many Western diets are hopelessly deficient in complex carbohydrate and dietary fibre and suffers from an excess of fat, salt, sugar and alcohol. None of these problems will be cured by even the most expensive vitamins.

A diet which contains foods such as wholegrains, breads, fruits and vegetables plus seafoods or poultry or lean meat or legumes, and some dairy products (preferably low fat) is almost certainly going to contain sufficient quantities of vitamins. Problems only arise if these foods are overcooked or are old and wilted. Those who choose to drink large quantities of alcohol or to live on a diet of fatty, sugary or highly salted processed foods can be assured that the alcohol, fat or salt will damage their livers, arteries, heart and kidneys long before they feel the effects of vitamins deficiency. Taking vitamins will not put off the day of reckoning. The only possible exception to this is for alcoholics who suffer real vitamin deficiencies. The provision of thiamin for these people can delay deterioration in brain cells.

Those who follow unbalanced slimming diets and anyone who has anorexia or vomits frequently after binge eating will need vitamin supplements. The vitamins won't solve the basic problem, but they will be necessary. Well-balanced slimming diets (see chapter 11) do not require extra vitamins.

Multi-vitamin preparations are unlikely to do any damage. However, many of the multi-vitamins currently available are quite unbalanced. A close examination of their contents reveals that some brands may have many times the recommended daily intake of some vitamins and only a minute fraction of the body's requirements for others. A few of the newer supplements have a better balance of vitamins in line with the recommended daily intakes as shown in Appendix 1g. If you are using a multi-vitamin, check out the quantities of the ingredients present against your daily needs.

A major problem with vitamin supplements is a lack of proper testing. With those pills containing moderate quantities of vitamins, testing is not needed. For the mega–dose vitamins, however, the same type of rigorous testing which must be applied to drugs should be mandatory. At present, most vitamins can be freely sold in drug-like quantities with no tests of their effects ever being required. This can, and does, cause health problems. Just because a substance is safe in small doses does not mean that more is better. There is no safe substance, only safe amounts.

Taking mega–doses of vitamins will achieve a vitamin-enriched sewerage; it may also damage some of the more delicate parts of the body. The body can become so used to excessive doses of vitamins that a drop in the flood can actually produce deficiency symptoms. Once addicted to high-dose supplements, the body may thus become dependent on a continued high level. To add insult to injury, taking large quantities of one vitamin (or mineral) may increase or decrease your need for other nutrients. Thus vitamins can often lead to an imbalance in the diet: the very thing they are advertised to correct.

We cannot make a blanket statement that vitamin supplements are either good or bad. It depends on the particular vitamin (or combination of vitamins), the level of the dose and whether or not the recipient really needs a supplement. There are people who must take particualr drugs which alter their requirements for vitamins. Supplements are often essential in such circumstances. However, we can state that:

- vitamin supplements do *not* provide balance to a poorly selected diet;
- vitamins *are* easily obtainable from foods;
- mega-doses of vitamins are entirely unnatural and should be subjected to rigorous testing before being peddled to a nutritionally illiterate public.

Let's take a look at the specific vitamins, see why they are important, how much you should be having, and where to find them in the food supply. We will also examine some of the myths associated with various vitamins.

VITAMIN A

This fat-soluble vitamin (properly known as retinol) comes from two sources:

1 Vitamin A itself occurs in foods such as liver and dairy products.
2 Beta–carotene, found in foods such as carrots, green and orange vegetables and fruits, is converted into vitamin A in the cells lining the intestine. The major part of our vitamin A usually comes from carotene.

Why is it important?

As children, we were told to eat carrots so that we could see in the dark. The reasoning behind this childhood admonition is that vitamin A is essential to make visual purple which enables the eye to adapt to dim light. A lack of vitamin A is the major cause of blindness throughout the world. It occurs in Australia in some malnourished Aboriginal children.

Vitamin A also helps to keep the linings of various membranes in the body in a healthy condition. This makes it valuable in preventing infection. In addition, vitamin A is essential for growth and normal reproduction, and for healthy skin.

Recently, vitamin A has generated interest for its possible preven-

122

tive role against cancer. Studies of cigarette smokers showed that those with the greatest intake of green and orange vegetables (potent suppliers of carotene) had some degree of protection from cancer. Whether it is actually the carotene in these foods, or some other factor, is still not known. The latest research suggests that it may be some of the other carotenoids (substances related to carotene) which provide the protection. Whatever the substance, it seems that you must actually eat the vegetables to gain the protection. Taking pills does not have the same value.

Other studies have shown that people with cancer tend to have lower than normal levels of vitamin A in their blood. Whether this occurs before or after the development of the cancer is not yet understood. However, it is known that the amount of vitamin A in the blood is related to more than the quantity of the vitamin A in the diet. Vitamin A is attached to a special protein in the blood and a limit of this will decrease the level of vitamin A.

How much do you need?

Adults need 750 micrograms of vitamin A (or retinol equivalents) a day. Children need lower quantities, as shown in Appendix 1g.

Each microgram of beta–carotene has the potency of one sixth of a microgram of the pre–formed vitamin A. Retinol equivalents are calculated by adding up the vitamin A values in foods plus one sixth of the carotene content.

Some people still refer to vitamin A in international units (IU). This terminology did not take into account the absorption of different forms of vitamin A and was phased out in 1974. One might question the update of knowledge of those who still quote vitamin A in these terms! To convert international units of vitamin A to micrograms of vitamin A (or retinol equivalents), divide by 3.33. (If the vitamin A comes from beta–carotene, divide the IU by 10.)

What happens if you lack vitamin A?

The effects of vitamin A deficiency include a hardening of the membranes in the eye and an increased susceptibility to infection.

What happens if you have too much?

If you are deficient in vitamin A, extra quantities of the vitamin will increase blood levels. But once you have exceeded the body's needs and the vitamin A-carrying protein has its full load, excess vitamin A piles up in the liver. Some of this can enter the blood and is quite toxic (that's why the body has a special protein to carry it around). It is therefore unwise to take excessive amounts of vitamin A: overzealous vitamin takers have died.

123

Women taking oral contraceptives have higher levels of vitamin A in the blood and it is inadvisable for them to take supplements.

The first effects of a toxicity of vitamin A include fatigue, irritability, dry skin, loss of appetite, vomiting, hair loss, headaches and pains in the bones.

Acute vitamin A poisoning will occur with a dose of 100 000 to 600 000 micrograms. Taking mega-doses of 10 000 to 50 000 micrograms a day over a period of months is also quite toxic.

Where do you find it?

The richest source of vitamin A is polar bear liver. With 50 000 to 100 000 micrograms in a 100-gram portion, it has been responsible for vitamin A poisoning.

Vitamin A is found in cod liver oil, liver, milk, cheese, butter, eggs and some fish and is added to some margarines. It is not in low-fat milk and this is the major reason why low-fat milk is not recommended for infants until they are old enough to eat a range of other foods to supply vitamin A or carotene.

Carotene occurs in all orange, yellow and green fruits and vegetables. The richest sources are carrots, yellow sweet potatoes (kumera), spinach, rockmelon, broccoli, mangoes, apricots, pumpkin, lettuce (especially the dark green outer leaves), watercress, tomatoes, peaches, prunes, parsley, Brussels sprouts, cabbage and capsicums. Just one medium-size carrot will contribute enough vitamin A for about three days.

Other points

Vitamin A interacts with vitamin E and also with zinc, iron and protein. Vitamin E helps to protect us from the toxicity of vitamin A. Vitamin A deficiency worsens the effects of a lack of iron or zinc. This is of importance for those suffering malnutrition.

VITAMIN B

The vitamin B–complex consists of eight separate vitamins. Each of these is water-soluble and some are easily lost when foods are heated. Food manufacturers may replace some of the vitamins lost during processing, for example thiamin, riboflavin and niacin are added to breakfast cereals although the other lost vitamins are not.

Originally the B–complex vitamins were called B_1, B_2, B_3, etc. However, some of the compounds originally thought to be members of the complex were subsequently found not to be true vitamins. Much of the numbering system has now been abandoned and the proper names are used instead. Table 10:1 lists the major points names are used instead. Table 10:1 lists the major points about the B-complex vitamin. It can be found at the end of the chapter.

VITAMIN C

Also called ascorbic acid, this is the most widely used vitamin because of its supposed ability to cure the common cold.

Why is it important?

Vitamin C is essential for the formation of connective tissue between cells. It forms a cementing type of material which holds cells together and keeps various body organs apart. It is important for healthy skin, mucous membranes, muscles, capillaries, bones and teeth. Vitamin C is also important in the formation of chemicals in the brain which control mood.

The importance of vitamin C has been known for centuries. Captain James Cook gave his crew sprouted wheat and limes to prevent scurvy, a well-known condition among sailors deprived of fresh fruit and vegetables for long periods. Yet, even as recently as the early part of this century, Scott's expedition to the South Pole ended in tragedy as frost bite took its toll on a party which had neglected to take any source of vitamin C.

The popularity of vitamin C gained a boost when several studies reported that it was protective against the common cold. Studies which compared the effects of vitamin C with a placebo (dummy pill) have since found that the vitamin does not reduce the number of colds although it does reduce the duration from just over six days to five days.

More success has been found with vitamin C's ability to prevent the formation of some cancer-producing substances. Nitrates are chemical compounds used to cure and control bacterial growth in meats such as bacon, hams and sausages. When combined with amines (substances which come from the amino acids in proteins) plus bacteria, the nitrates can form cancer–causing chemicals called nitrosamines. Vitamin C prevents their formation. It thus makes good sense to eat a food containing vitamin C with one containing nitrates. For examples, bacon is best eaten with tomatoes, ham with pineapple or some other fruit, and sausages with vegetables or followed by fresh fruit.

Vitamin C may also be involved in protection against heart disease, although there are still conflicting results to be resolved. Vitamin C is involved in the manufacture of the body's cholesterol and may affect its excretion. However, vitamin C also influences the way the body uses zinc and copper and it may be via these minerals that the vitamin protects the arteries.

How much do you need?

The body's normal stores of vitamin C can last for approximately three weeks. However, since some vitamin C is lost each day, it is important to replace it regularly. Most animals make their own vitamin C; it is only humans, guinea pigs and monkeys who must obtain it from the diet.

The Recommended Daily Intake is 30 milligrams per day for adults and children. During pregnancy and lactation, this increases to 60 milligrams per day.

The body's tissues will be saturated with vitamin C with a daily intake of about 100 milligrams per day and there is no point in taking the massive doses which are so commonly used. Cigarette smoking increases the need for vitamin C and smokers may need 100 to 130 milligrams per day to produce saturation of the body tissues.

Contrary to popular belief, athletes do not need extra vitamin C. Some early studies suggested that the muscles in the fingers took longer to become fatigued when extra vitamin C was taken. However, better-controlled studies have shown that vitamin C does not affect muscle fatigue or prevent stiffness after exercise.

Claims are also made that vitamin C will slow down the ageing process and will help to cure cancer. These claims are not supported by properly controlled medical research. One study has shown that guinea pigs, which cannot make their own vitamin C, will have a reduced life span if given large doses of the vitamin.

Vitamin C is found in high concentration in the adrenal glands which are responsible for making hormones to help us to cope with various stresses. Some people claim that extra vitamin C will increase the ability to cope with stress. This theory falls into the category of assuming a car will run better if the petrol tank is overflowing. Enough is enough.

What happens if you lack vitamin C?

A complete lack of vitamin C will cause scurvy with its associated infections. Before reaching this stage, vitamin C deficiency produces bleeding gums, joint pains, bruising, wounds which do not heal, fatigue and muscular weakness.

What happens if you have too much?

Excessive amounts of vitamin C come from tablets or ascorbic acid powder, not from food. The body can tolerate quite large amounts of vitamin C. However, once the intake is too high, the excess is not absorbed from the intestine and passes from the blood to the kidneys for excretion in urine.

The first noticeable symptom of vitamin C overload is diarrhoea. Some vitamin salespeople maintain that you know you are having sufficient vitamin C when diarrhoea begins. This is absurd and indicates that the intestine may be unable to absorb other nutrients.

With an intake of vitamin C of more than 4000 milligrams a day, more uric and oxalic acids are excreted from the kidneys and pose a possible risk of kidney stones.

High levels of vitamin C have also been shown to cause rebound scurvy when discontinued. This has occurred in babies born to women taking high doses of vitamin C. Having been used to these excessive quantities, the baby's body has come to regard them as normal.

Too much vitamin C may also cause excessive amounts of iron to be absorbed and may increase the absorption of other, undesirable minerals such as mercury.

If you are tempted to take high doses of vitamin C, you should also be aware that it will alter the effect of aspirin, anti–depressants and drugs which control the thickness of blood. It may also interfere with fertility or induce a condition which resembles diabetes.

For all these reasons, it seems crazy to take massive doses of vitamin C when the only proven benefit is that it reduces a cold by one day.

Where do you find it?

Vitamin C is found in breast milk and in fruits and vegetables. It is easily lost when fruits and vegetables are squashed, stored at room temperature for long periods, or cooked. Some raw fruits and vegetables should be eaten each day. Vegetables which are microwaved, steamed or stir fried will lose less vitamin C than those which are boiled in a large quantity of water. Overcooking and the old habit of adding bicarbonate of soda to make vegetables bright green also increase the loss of vitamin C.

Among fruits and vegetables, the best sources of vitamin C are: guavas, broccoli, capsicums, papaws, Brussels sprouts, strawberries, oranges, rockmelons, mangoes, kiwifruit, grapefruit, cauliflower, cabbage, lychees, custard apples, lemons, gooseberries, raspberries, pineapples, tomatoes, watercress and spinach. An average serve of any of these foods will supply more than the day's needs.

Some vitamin C is also found in blackberries, asparagus, avocado, potatoes, peas, parsley and apples.

To preserve the vitamin C in these foods, try to:

- Choose products in good condition (no wilting, bruising).
- Keep products refrigerated.

127

- Prepare as close to eating time as possible.
- Eat raw or cook by microwave, steam or stir fry.
- Finish cooking when vegetables are barely tender.
- Avoid leaving vegetables soaking in water.
- Use a microwave if re-heating is necessary.

Frozen vegetables retain much of their vitamin C, but should not be thawed before cooking.

VITAMIN D

This is one vitamin which need not concern those who live in a sunny climate. A form of Vitamin D is made when ultraviolet rays of sunlight act on a substance in the skin. This substance is then converted to another form of vitamin D in the liver and finally to a third form in the kidneys. With sunlight available for so much of the year, vitamin D deficiency is rare in Australia, for example. Problems can occur when there is a disorder of the liver or kidneys so that the most potent forms of vitamin D are not made, and in elderly people whose clothing covers all their skin.

Why is it important?

Vitamin D is essential for calcium and phosphorus to be absorbed into bones. You can eat as much calcium as you like, but if there is no vitamin D present, the calcium will not be absorbed. For people with very low intakes of calcium, vitamin D will increase the percentage of the calcium which is taken up by the bones.

How much do you need?

We cannot estimate the amount of vitamin D made by the action of sunlight on the skin. However, a safe estimate is 5 micrograms a day for adults and 10 micrograms for children. Larger doses are not advisable.

What happens if you lack vitamin D?

A deficiency of vitamin D leads to misshapen bones. In children, the disorder is known as rickets. It occurs in countries where the weather is so cold that skin is not exposed to sunlight. In adults, a deficiency of vitamin D also causes weakening of the bones leading to a disease called osteomalacia. It is characterised by bone pain and spasms in the muscles attached to bones.

What happens if you have too much?

Vitamin D is quite toxic and there have been many cases of overzealous people suffering from vitamin D poisoning. With excessive doses of vitamin D (from tablets or cod liver oil), too much calcium is absorbed into the blood and some is deposited in soft tissues. Nerves, muscles, the spleen and the kidneys can become hard and calcified. Initial symptoms include headache, loss of appetite and vomiting, followed by kidney stones, increased blood pressure and problems with lung function.

Excess vitamin D is a problem since the quantities which cause toxicity are quite low. Taking as little as five times the normal requirement can be dangerous. Sunlight does not produce excess vitamin D because the tanning of the skin shuts off the process whereby the vitamin D substances are made. Excess comes from supplements, or from foods which are particularly rich in vitamin D, such as cod liver oil.

The problems of excess vitamin D are much greater in countries where various foods, such as infant foods, have added vitamin D. While this supplementation is important in areas where the weather is very cold, it must be strictly controlled. Food legislation now governs the quantities which can be added, yet many parents maintain the tradition of feeding their children supplements of cod liver oil.

Where do you find it?

Food sources of vitamin D are kippers, herring, mackerel, salmon, sardines, tuna, margarine, liver, milk, butter and cheese.

Cod liver oil is the richest source of vitamin D. With more than 200 micrograms of vitamin D per 100 millilitres, just one teaspoon of cod liver oil can supply a child's entire needs for the day. In sunny climates, cod liver oil is unnecessary and should be avoided except for those people who cannot go out into sunshine.

VITAMIN E

Vitamin E is a collection of substances known as tocopherols. The different members of this family have varying levels of potency for humans, with alpha–tocopherol being the most important.

For some years, it was difficult to find anyone with a deficiency of vitamin E so the condition could be studied. Some vitamin sellers made vitamin E the star of all vitamins, claiming that it would cure everything from heart disease to impotence to ulcers. For a time, vitamin E became trendy.

129

Why is it important?

Vitamin E is an antioxidant which functions with the mineral selenium to protect cells from the damaging effects of oxygen radicals. A deficiency of either the vitamin or the mineral allows damage to cell membranes. Polyunsaturated fats are especially in need of protection since oxygen will cause them to break down and to form undesirable compounds which may damage membranes around cells. Vitamin E may also offer protection against other toxic chemicals and is involved in the formation of haemoglobin, the red pigment which carries oxygen in the blood.

Vitamin E also gives protection against various toxic chemical substances. For example, it is protective against ozone and nitrous oxide. Since these substances cause a breakdown in the fat in cell membranes, vitamin E probably acts as an antioxidant and prevents damage to the membrane.

In some animals vitamin E has additional functions. Some male animals, for example, suffer from atrophy of the testicles when they are deficient in vitamin E. An extrapolation of this fact has led to enormous sales of vitamin E among humans who hope to achieve super sexual prowess with the aid of vitamin E supplements. No such effects have ever been shown in humans.

Vitamin E is a most important vitamin but it is not a miraculous youth preserver which will provide radiant skin, a healthy heart, strong muscles, prevention from cancer and a raging sex life: these are all claims which are sometimes made for it.

How much do you need?

The quantity of vitamin E required depends on the amount of polyunsaturated fat eaten. The more oils and polyunsaturated fats consumed, the greater the vitamin E requirement. This does not mean that chips cooked in oil should be followed by a vitamin E capsule. Many polyunsaturated fats are also good sources of vitamin E: a ready-made partnership.

It is generally recommended that an intake of 10 to 20 milligrams of vitamin E per day will meet an adult's needs, assuming that polyunsaturated fats make up around 10 per cent of the diet. Most people eat less of these fats than that, and so such an amount will be ample. For those who would like more precise information, it is recommended that 0.4 milligrams of vitamin E be consumed for every gram of polyunsaturated fatty acid in the diet.

What happens if you lack vitamin E?

A deficiency of vitamin E has been seen in premature babies and occasionally in those who have had extensive gastrointestinal disorders which prevent the absorption of any fat. A lack of vitamin E causes red blood cells to break down more easily than normal. Nerve cells and muscle fibres also suffer. Vitamin E deficiency is rare as there is a considerable amount stored in the body.

What happens if you have too much?

Vitamin E does not seem to be very toxic to humans. At doses of 300 milligrams per day, some nausea and gastric upsets occur. In animals, excessive vitamin E has been shown to alter the action of the thyroid gland and to prevent normal growth. Large doses also prevent vitamin D from fulfilling its normal function and may induce a deficiency of vitamin K. One study found that 800 to 1200 milligrams of vitamin E prevented the normal clotting of blood. As with all vitamins, it is preferable not to overdo the amount of vitamin E coming from supplements.

Where do you find it?

Vitamin E is widely distributed in foods. The best sources are wheatgerm oil, sunflower oil, safflower oil, cottonseed oil, hazelnuts, almonds, wheatgerm, sunflower seeds, pepitas, (pumpkin seeds), blackberries, canned tuna, sweet potato, avocado, peanuts, Brazil nuts, lobster, asparagus, salmon, peanut butter, spinach, tomatoes, wholegrain cereals, vegetable margarines, broccoli, sweetcorn, Brussels sprouts, oysters, fish, legumes, dairy products and meats.

VITAMIN K

This fat-soluble vitamin was discovered in the 1930s and consists of a number of different substances. Studies on the vitamin have been difficult since much of our vitamin K is made by bacteria in the intestine.

Why is it important?

Vitamin K helps to form blood clots. These are important so that we do not continue to bleed after injury. Vitamin K may also be involved in the formation of protein substances in the bones and kidneys.

How much do you need?

Requirements for vitamin K are estimated to be 70 to 140 micrograms a day for adults, 15 to 100 micrograms a day for adolescents and 10 to 20 micrograms a day for children. It is estimated that about half of our vitamin K is made in the intestine.

What happens if you lack vitamin K?

Vitamin K deficiency sometimes occurs in newborn babies. At birth there are no bacteria in the intestine and so no vitamin K is manufactured. If insufficient vitamin K has passed from mother to the foetus, the child may develop haemorrhages and these can affect such vital organs as the brain. For most babies, breast milk supplies vitamin K.

In adults, vitamin K deficiency may occur after a prolonged course of antibiotics or in any disease in which fats cannot be absorbed.

Without sufficient vitamin K, bleeding time is extended and this may lead to severe blood loss and anaemia. It may occur if the liver is damaged by alcohol.

What happens if you have too much?

Many times the daily requirements can be consumed without any apparent harm. Synthetic forms of vitamin K, however, can be toxic in large doses.

Where do you find it?

Healthy bacteria living and multiplying in the intestine make much of our vitamin K.

Among foods, the best sources include spinach, lettuce, soya beans, cauliflower, cabbage, broccoli, liver, mushrooms, peas, beans, potatoes and carrots. Meats and dairy products contain small quantities, but fruits and cereals have little vitamin K.

Other points

The fact that vitamin K is intimately concerned with normal clotting of blood means that it will interact with drugs which are given to 'thin' the blood. If there is a danger of blood clotting too easily (for example, where someone has thrombosis or a clot in an artery), drugs are given to prevent the blood from clotting. The dose of an anti–clotting drug (such as warfarin) will be established for a particular person. Taking vitamin K or changing the usual amount of vitamin K–rich foods such as vegetables can alter the dose of the drug required and could lead either to unusual bleeding or clotting.

Table 10.1 The B-complex vitamins

Why it is important	How much is needed	Deficiency symptoms	What about excess?	Where it is found	Other points
		Thiamin (B$_1$)			
Needed for carbo-hydrates to be used in the body. Also vital for the brain, nervous system, digestive system and the heart.	Women 0.8–1.1 mg/day Men 0.9–1.3 mg/day Pregnancy 1.0 mg/day Lactation 1.1 mg/day	Muscle weakness, loss of limb function, loss of memory and appe-tite. Occurs in alcoholics, and can occur in those who eat a lot of sugar or fat, but few nutritious foods.	Not generally dangerous unless a large dose is injected.	Pork, kidney, liver, bread (especially wholemeal), yeast extract, legumes, peas, wholegrain cereals, lean meat, chicken, fish. Some is de-stroyed by heat. Microwaves are less destructive.	High levels of thiamin have been noted in cases of cot death.
		Riboflavin (B$_2$)			
Needed for the body to use proteins. Also needed by the thyroid gland, and for healthy skin and normal tissue repair.	Women 1.3 mg/day Men 1.6 mg/day Pregnancy 1.6 mg/day Lactation 1.8 mg/day	Dermatitis and skin lesions, lowered resistance to infection and possibly certain types of cancer.	Only massive doses (500 mg/kg) would damage the kidneys and cause death. Excess amounts are quickly lost in urine, which appears bright yellow–green.	Liver, kidney, milk, yeast ex-tract, cheese, yoghurt, al-monds, breakfast cereals, mush-rooms, chicken, lean meat, eggs. Little is lost in cooking.	Pasteurisa-tion of milk causes a loss of 5%; four hours of sun-light results in 70% loss.
		Niacin (B$_3$)			
Needed for the body to use pro-teins, carbohy-drates and fats. Essential for healthy skin. Can be made from an amino acid in protein foods.	Women 10–14 mg/day Men 14–20 mg/day Pregnancy 14–16 mg/day Lactation 17–19 mg/day	Dermatitis of skin exposed to sun, weakness, diar-rhoea, mental depression.	Flushing and itchiness of the skin, increased use of glycogen from muscles, disturbance to heart rhythm, dizziness. May cause gout or diabetes.	Liver, tuna, chicken, fish, salmon, kidney, lean meat, wholemeal bread, mushrooms, yeast extract, breakfast cereals, legumes, dried fruits, potato. Lost if foods are overcooked.	Sometimes promoted as a cure for schizoph-renia but controlled tests have not shown benefits.
		Pyridoxine (B$_6$)			
Needed for the body to use pro-tein. Also helps in formation of haemoglobin in blood.	Women 0.9–1.4 mg/day Men 1.3–1.9 mg/day Pregnancy 1.0–1.5 mg/day Lactation 1.6–2.2 mg/day	Mental depression, dermatitis of the face, weight loss, irritability, weakness.	Continually taking doses of several hundred milli-grams can harm nerve endings in fingers and toes. Dependence on continued high dose occurs. Avoid taking more than 25 mg/day.	Liver, kidney, pork, bananas, lentils, avocado, fish, eggs, turkey, chicken, tuna, salmon, walnuts, lean meat, pota-toes, wheatgerm, legumes. Lost at very high cooking temperatures.	The com-mon idea that B$_6$ will cure symptoms of pre–men-strual syn-drome has led many women to take high doses.

Table 10.1 The B-complex vitamins — continued

Why it is important	How much is needed	Deficiency symptoms	What about excess?	Where it is found	Other points
Essential for red blood cells and nerve cells. Also needed to make DNA. Body stores will last for 3–6 years.	Women and Men 2.0 mg/day Pregnancy 3.0 mg/day Lactation 2.5 mg/day	**Cyanocobalamin (B$_{12}$)** Pernicious anaemia, abnormal pigmentation of the skin. Usually develops because the B$_{12}$ cannot be absorbed. Occasionally seen in strict vegetarians. B$_{12}$ deficiency masks folate deficiency	No known effect as the excess does not seem to be absorbed. Those who are deficient generally need B$_{12}$ injections.	Liver and kidney are by far the richest sources. Also in oysters, tuna, fish, meat, chicken, eggs, milk, cheese and yoghurt. Mushrooms and fermented soya products may contain some. Only small losses with cooking.	B$_{12}$ was only isolated 40 years ago.
Needed for protein synthesis, by red blood cells and to make DNA. Linked with B$_{12}$.	Women and Men 200 mcg/day Pregnancy 400 mcg/day Lactation 300–350 mcg/day	**Folate** Irritability, insomnia, anaemia in which red blood cells do not mature. Probably the most common vitamin deficiency.	High doses may produce gastro-intestinal disturbances. More than 400 mcg/day may mask B$_{12}$ deficiency.	Liver is extremely rich. Also in green vegetables (endive, broccoli, spinach, Brussels sprouts), avocado, peanuts, peas, wholemeal bread, grains. Large losses if vegetables are boiled. Try to include some raw vegetables.	Folate interacts with some drugs. Alcohol, anti-malarial drugs and some anti-cancer drugs may cause folate deficiency. If folate is given to epileptics on anti-convulsants, fits sometimes increase.
Needed to make fatty acids, cholesterol and haemoglobin. Also important in nerves and muscles.	Women and Men 4–7 mg/day Pregnancy and Lactation 20 mg/day	**Pantothenic acid** Abdominal pains, vomiting, insomnia, personality changes, leg cramps, diarrhoea. Deficiency is rare, but may occur with ulcerative colitis.	High doses seem useless but fairly innocuous. Megadoses may cause diarrhoea.	Liver and yeast very rich. Also in kidney, watermelon, chicken, pork, lentils, peanuts, avocado, turkey, lean meat, eggs, milk and wholemeal bread. Lost if foods are overcooked or reheated.	Some animals' hair turns grey with a lack of pantothenic acid, but this is not the cause of grey hair in humans.

Table 10.1   The B-complex vitamins — continued

Why it is important	How much is needed	Deficiency symptoms	What about excess?	Where it is found	Other points
		Biotin			
Needed to make fatty acids and to produce glucose. Important for healthy skin and hair.	Usually made by bacteria in the intestine, so dietary requirement is difficult to establish. Women and Men 100–200 mcg/day	May cause a drop in blood glucose. Dry skin, loss of body hair, loss of appetite, high blood cholesterol, depression. May occur if large quantities of raw egg white (10 eggs per day) are eaten or with prolonged use of antibiotics which kill the good bacteria which normally make biotin.	No adverse effects with doses of 5000 to 10 000 mcg given to infants with a rare form of dermatitis. In animals, high doses may stop reproduction.	Liver and kidney very rich. Also in yeast, eggs, oats, oysters, legumes, milk, rice bran, chicken, meat, fish, avocado. Raw egg white has a substance, avidin, which destroys biotin. Avidin is killed by cooking egg whites.	Biotin is often missing from multi–vitamins, but may be needed with prolonged use of anti–biotics. A lack has been linked with cot death, but more research is needed.

The tables above give the recommended intakes for Australians. In Britain no recommended amounts have been set for B-complex vitamins other than Thiamin and Riboflavin.

135

11

Weight:
How do you get it right?

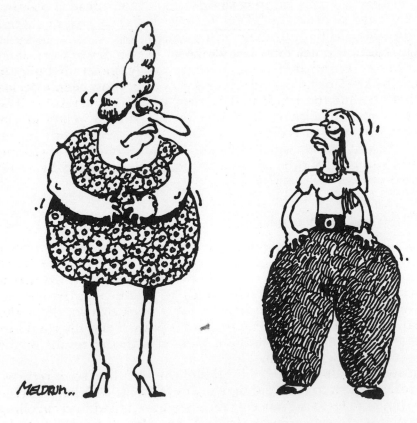

DIETING is said to be the most popular indoor sport of women. There is no doubt that many women and an increasing number of men seek out the latest diet. As publishers are aware, the latest diet will move women's magazines, and diet books make best sellers. By some quirk of reasoning, the crazier the diet, the more likely it is to attract followers.

Why diets don't work

With almost 50 per cent of men and women over forty carrying excess body fat, it's hardly surprising that dieting is so popular. The problem is that most diets simply do not work, at least not in the long term. In fact, many diets actually make people fat. If that notion sounds ridiculous, you only need to talk to overweight people to find that those who have tried dozens of diets have found themselves becoming steadily fatter. Sure, the weight drops initially, but then it all comes back, usually with a few bonus kilos. But instead of blaming the diet, most overweight people believe that their lack of success has something to do with their own metabolism.

The crush on crazy diets is a symptom of our desire for instant gratification. Excess body weight comes slowly, generally building up, kilo by kilo, over a period of years. But once most people decide it's time to shift the resident flab, they want instant results. The popular diets capitalise on the desire for fast painless weight loss by providing it! You've seen the captions: 'Lose ten pounds in ten days!', 'Fastest, easiest weight loss ever!', 'Eat as much as you want, and still lose weight!', and so on. If they were all so good, why would we need so many of them?

Why diets appear to work

It is quite possible to manipulate the diet to cause a fast loss of body weight. About two-thirds of the body's weight is water. This can fluctuate by several kilos if the carbohydrate content of the diet is suddenly reduced. This is the basis of most popular weight-reduction diets. You follow the diet for a week or two, the scales appear to record great success, the diet is praised and the would-be slimmer feels somewhat tired, but pleased with the results of the week or two of deprivation.

But such 'results' are short-lived and the lost fluid soon returns. The scales return to their old figure, or even a little higher, and the poor slimmers feel that, once again, they have failed in controlling their diet and body weight. In fact, the diet 'worked' only by temporarily removing fluid.

The idea that overweight people have accumulated too much   **137** fluid is popular, but incorrect. Fat has a much lower content of water than muscle and those who are too fat actually have a lower percentage of body weight as water than those who are lean. It may be more socially acceptable to say that you are heavy because of fluid retention, but it is rarely correct.

One exception to this occurs in women who retain extra fluid just before their menstrual period. At such times, hormonal changes cause extra sodium to be retained in the tissues and this, in turn, holds some extra water, sometimes as much as two kilograms extra. The way to prevent this occurring is to drink more water. This may sound like adding insult to injury, but extra water will flush out the sodium which is causing the fluid retention. Eating less salt will also help. Once the period begins, the hormones again alter and the extra water will be lost. A few women find that they also retain some extra fluid at the time of ovulation, mid-way through the menstrual cycle. Drinking extra water and eating less salt will again correct this situation. In general, however, fluid retention is not a cause of excess weight. The real problem in overweight people is too much body fat.

Fast weight loss is only achieved by depriving the body of some of its normal fluid content. With most of these diets, loss of body fat is minimal. Whenever weight loss occurs at a rate of more than about a kilogram a week, you can be fairly certain that you are losing fluid rather than fat. Don't be surprised when the lost fluid returns.

By going thirsty or having a sauna and not replacing the lost fluids, you can also reduce fluid. Such actions are foolish since the kidneys and other organs need water to function at peak performance.

Those who are trying to exercise will also find their performance severely affected by anything which reduces the normal content of water in the body. Muscle cells need plenty of water. In spite of the absurdity, an amazing collection of diets exist which 'work' by depriving the body of some of its vitally important fluid.

Other diets go for the 'have your cake and eat it too' approach. Some popular food is singled out and taken as the 'name' for the diet. And so we have 'The Banana Diet', 'The Watermelon Diet', 'The Spaghetti Diet', 'The Egg Diet', 'The Drinking Man's Diet' or some other title designed to make people think that they can have their favourite or 'forbidden' food and still lose weight. The fine print of the diet usually shows the reality. Either you can eat as much of that particular food as you like, but nothing else, or there are restrictions on the usual accompaniments to such foods. One popular diet, for example, says that you can have as much pasta as you like, but closer inspection reveals that the pasta must be eaten completely on its own and, on 'pasta days', no other food may be eaten. Under such circumstances, the quantity of pasta eaten will be minimal, at least after the first day or two! The idea behind single-food diets is that few people can eat very much of any one food and so the total amount of kilojoules actually consumed drops.

The same idea pervades the type of diet which says that you can have as much fat and protein as you like, but no carbohydrate foods. It may sound great to be told that you can eat loads of meat, butter, cream and bacon, but in reality there is a limit to how much cream or butter you can eat when everything you would normally have with them is forbidden.

The principle behind the fast weight-loss diets

Almost all popular diets work on a principle which is well known to biochemists. By restricting the intake of carbohydrate foods, the body is forced to use its muscle stores of carbohydrate or glycogen. Since every gram of glycogen in muscles is stored with 2.7 grams of water, the loss of muscle glycogen is accompanied by a large loss of water from the body. This shows up on the scales as a loss of weight and brings initial joy to the heart of the slimmer. Sadly, though, it is not fat which is being lost, but glycogen and water. Once you go back to eating even a moderate diet, the body replaces its glycogen, and the normal water which goes with it. As many athletes who practise the technique of carbohydrate loading are aware, the initial deprivation of carbohydrate followed by re-feeding means that the body stores a little more glycogen than normal. After the diet, body weight can actually increase to a level higher than before the diet.

Even worse, however, is the fact that a low-carbohydrate diet forces the body to break down some of its muscle, or lean tissue. This occurs because the body must maintain a certain level of glucose in the blood. The brain can function only with glucose as its energy source: it cannot run on fat. Since it is biochemically impossible for body fat to be broken down to glucose, inadequate carbohydrate in the diet means that the body will be forced to break down some of its lean tissue to replenish the supply of glucose in the blood. This is a clever adaptation to survival during starvation, but it can be disastrous for future weight control.

Body fat uses up few kilojoules: it is metabolically inactive. Muscle or lean tissue, on the other hand, uses up quite a bit of energy. To explain this further, let us consider the example of two men, both 180 centimetres tall and weighing 72 kilograms. One of our men is an athlete and has well-developed muscles, the other has very little physical activity to cause muscle growth and more of his body is fat. If we were to measure the amount of energy burned up by the two men, we would find that the guy with the most muscle would be

139

burning up far more kilojoules, even when he was sitting still. He would therefore be able to eat more food without gaining weight than our man with less lean tissue, even though both were the same height and weight. Both men will have similar metabolic rates per unit of lean tissue but the lean man has more lean tissue. Thus he uses more kilojoules in metabolism than the man with the same frame but less muscle.

Slimmers who follow a low-carbohydrate diet will lose some of their muscle or lean tissue with the result that they will need fewer kilojoules after the diet than they needed before. The net result of the popular low-carbohydrate diets can be summarised as:

- an initial loss of body glycogen and water;
- followed by a regaining of glycogen and water;
- plus a net loss of lean tissue;
- and, consequently, a reduced need for kilojoules.

This was the theory behind the old 'no bread, no potatoes' advice which doctors gave their patients. It is also the idea behind most of the gimmicky weight-loss diets which abound. Even though the diet may promise you 'bananas, pasta, icecream' or whatever, in practice it is likely to be a low-carbohydrate diet designed for quick water loss. Fat loss will be minimal and post–diet weight gain is almost inevitable.

After a dozen or so diets, the loss of lean body tissue can be sufficient for even a moderate food intake to make a person fat. Some overweight people obviously eat and drink a lot of high-kilojoule foods. But some do not. This latter group once ate more food than was needed and gained extra fat. Then they became chronic dieters and reduced their kilojoule needs so far that even small amounts of food became fattening. Dieting actually made them fat.

Fortunately, many people are discovering the stupidity of gimmick diets and are realising that the only way to lose weight is to consider both the kilojoules coming *into* the body and those being *used* by the body for metabolism and physical activity. By cutting back too far on what you eat you simply reduce the body's output in metabolism and make it difficult to feel energetic enough to exercise. It is important to have sufficient kilojoules coming from complex carbohydrate so that you *can* carry out an exercise programme. Muscles cannot function well without this vital fuel.

Fast weight loss is almost always followed by fast weight gain. Even if you are following a sensible eating and exercise programme, it is important that the loss of body fat should be gradual. Medical researchers have found that any sudden drop in body fat means that fat is being emptied out of the fat cells, but the cells stay there, ready to soak up their usual amount of fat at the first opportunity.

A slower fat loss may seem boring, but it can help fat cells to gradually lose their fat content and shrivel up. Early ideas that fat cells only develop in infancy and at puberty have been shown to be incorrect. Using much more sophisticated equipment, smaller fat cells can now be detected. It appears that fat cells can come or go throughout life, although the greatest rate of increase is likely to be in infancy and at puberty. Fat children have a high chance of becoming fat adults, but even thin children can develop extra fat cells as adults if they eat more food than their bodies need.

Weight

Who needs to lose weight: the 'apples' and 'pears' theory

Many people ignore the realities of health problems associated with excess fat while others who are not even overweight are constantly trying to lose their perfectly normal levels of body fat. In the majority of such cases, it is men who ignore their excess fat (even denying that they have any) while many normal-weight women become obsessed with weight loss. Some women spend most of their waking hours worrying about their supposed 'excess' fat deposits: many develop chronic eating disorders as a result.

Body fat is deposited in different ways, depending to some extent on your basic body shape, but also on your sex. Men tend to put down their fat around the waist. The much-displayed and affectionately regarded beer-gut is nothing but fat. Some women also deposit their excess flesh around the waist, but most find that it tends to accumulate more on the hips, tummy and thighs.

With excess body fat, we can basically divide people into two major categories: 'apples' and 'pears'. 'Apples' have their excess fat around the middle and on the upper body: they rarely have fat legs. 'Pears', on the other hand, tend to carry more of their fat on the hips, tummy and thighs. There are exceptions, but most overweight men fit the category of 'apples' while fat women tend to be 'pears'.

'Apples' have far more health risks associated with their excess fat than 'pears'. Fat around the waist and on the upper body increases the risk of diabetes, coronary heart disease, gallstones and high blood pressure. 'Pears' have little increased risk of these problems. Yet it is the 'pear'-shaped women who worry most about their excess body fat.

Few women measure up to the media 'ideal' body shape and the normal female body is somewhat 'pear'-shaped. Thus we have women, who are not overweight, who believe that their size and shape are wrong. One study, reported in an Australian consumers' magazine, found that 76 per cent of women at the lighter end of the healthy weight range wanted to be lighter still. Another study of 20-year-old female university students reported that 94 per cent thought

141

that they were too fat; very few were. Other studies have found that the majority of women are unhappy with their basic body shape.

Many men, on the other hand, refuse to accept that their expanding waistline is anything more than an occupational hazard. Some are quite proud of their 'beer-gut' and its affinity with the amber liquid. Others find an expanding girth takes up more 'space' and increases their feelings of importance. A small percentage of men who are a healthy weight want to be heavier, but most men are quite happy with their size and spend much less time agonising over it than women. In view of the 50 per cent of men who are overweight, and their predisposition to the 'apple' shape, this complacency is misplaced.

There are also men and women who are aware of their genuinely excessive levels of body fat who like to do something about it. If that fat is on the upper body, there are good medical reasons to be concerned.

What some women perceive as excess flesh is a normal female distribution of body fat. Female hormones dictate that there should be some fat stores on the hips and thighs. Researchers have found that female thigh fat is remarkably stable: something most women could have told them! During pregnancy, and, to an even greater degree, during lactation thigh fat is easily mobilised to provide extra kilojoules. Women seem to have stores of fat on the thighs to provide for their offspring should a famine occur. The survival of the species in past times could well have depended on female thighs! Since famines are no longer part of life in Western countries, and because the media often portray a female body with the thighs of an undeveloped 14 year old, many women starve themselves in an effort to remove their perfectly normal fat stores. If the woman is not fat in other areas of her body, she should accept that her thigh fat will not budge unless she becomes so thin that her hormones no longer function properly and her periods cease.

The modern woman also suffers from the problem of a lack of physical activity. Exercise will increase the thigh muscle and hold the fat in place more firmly, giving the appearance of a firm thigh rather than a flabby thigh. Ironically, many women will not take the exercise which would improve the muscle tone on their thighs because they are worried that someone will see their thighs while they exercise!

We are all stuck with our basic body shape. Just as you cannot alter your height, neither can you turn a 'pear' shape into the upside-down 'pear'-shape which many women desire. A large 'pear' who loses weight will simply become a smaller 'pear'. A small 'pear' will become an even smaller 'pear' and this may emphasise the shape to an even greater extent.

Following a sensible eating and exercise pattern to remove excess body fat will cause a loss of fat from the whole body, and not only from selected areas. Just as you cannot ask your car to burn only the fuel in the top right-hand corner of its petrol tank, neither can you make your body use up only the fat on certain areas. We are stuck with our basic shape and the sooner most women can accept that fact, the happier and healthier we will be.

The health risks associated with excess body fat

Assuming that you are genuinely overweight, the health story is one of doom and gloom. The human body has been designed to operate efficiently without a heap of excess fat. When it is required to carry a heavy load, its basic machinery often fails and health problems result.

For every ten kilograms of excess fat, it has been estimated that there are 29 kilometres of extra blood vessels through which blood must be pumped. To make it worse, fat surrounding the heart makes pumping more difficult. So the heart and blood vessels do not like extra fat: it makes their job too demanding. Just as a tiny engine will not be able to move a bus around for too long, so the heart of an overweight person tends to give up sooner than normal. For the sake of your heart, it is preferable to be lean.

An overfat body is also likely to have large quantities of fat in the blood. This will lead to deposits of fatty material in blood vessels, narrowing their diameter. When the heart must continually pump against pressure, the arteries gradually become less elastic and blood pressure rises. For the sake of your blood pressure, it is preferable to be lean.

Insulin is a hormone produced in the body to enable glucose to pass from the blood into the body cells. An overfat body demands much more insulin. In the majority of cases of type II diabetes (that is, the kind which develops in adults), the production of insulin is insufficient because of excess weight. For the sake of your insulin production, it is preferable to be lean.

Gallstones are a common health problem in Western countries. They are related to a high-fat diet. Some thin people develop gallstones if too much of what they eat consists of fat. In general, though, gallstones are much more common among overweight people. For the sake of your gallbladder, it is preferable to be lean.

Certain types of cancer have now been linked with excess weight. Cancer of the bowel, and the hormone-dependent cancers of the breast, cervix and uterus, and, possibly, the prostate gland in men, are more common in the overweight. In older women, an increase in fatty tissue in the breasts produces oestrogen which may upset the hormone system. High levels of dietary fat, which easily produce excess weight, are particularly implicated in breast and prostate cancer. With bowel cancer, it is not yet clear whether it is excess weight, or the high-fat diet which produces it, which increases the risks. But it is clear that for protection against cancer, it is preferable to be lean.

Conditions such as arthritis and back and joint disorders are not caused by excess weight, but they do become worse if you are too fat. Increased weight stresses the joints and for their sake, it is preferable to be lean.

The greater the body weight, the higher the dose of anaesthetic required for surgical procedures. So if you need surgery, it is also preferable to be lean.

In fact, it is difficult to find any advantage in being overweight beyond a decreased likelihood of osteoporosis. Having to carry around excess weight will strengthen bones so that they are less likely to break. This is just as well, since any bone fractures which *do* occur will create greater difficulty in the overweight.

Without a doubt, it is better to be lean than fat. However, that does *not* mean that everyone needs to look rake-like. Extremes are usually foolish. The overweight certainly have a greater risk of health problems. So do those who are very underweight. Ideally, we need to keep weight within normal limits. Check the chart, Appendix 1h to see whether your weight is too high, too low or just about right.

The best way to lose excess weight

The best way to lose weight is not to get fat in the first place! So if you are slim, continue to exercise and to eat sensibly to stay that way. If you are already overweight, you need a sensible approach to diet and exercise. Fast weight-loss diets are not the answer. There is no point in attempting to lose weight unless you are prepared to accept a few facts. These are:

1   Body fat can only be lost slowly. Fast weight loss means that much of what you are losing is water and muscle. Content yourself with a weekly fat loss of 0.5 to 1 kilogram. To get some idea of how much fat this is, take a look at the contents of a tub or two of margarine. If you could lose that much fat each week, you would be achieving a lot.

2   There are no miracles! Give up hoping that someone will find a way to eat and drink as much as you like without gaining weight. There are no magic pills, supplements, drinks, biscuits, special fat-burning food combinations, passive exercise

machines, creams, special clothing or other paraphernalia which will melt away excess flab.

3   There is no way that you can go on a diet for a few weeks or months and then go back to your old habits. You need to be committed to a new life-long eating and exercise plan with meals and snacks made up of appropriate quantities of healthy foods. Before you despair, remember that no food need be completely banned and that healthy foods taste great. Once your body becomes used to high-quality, nutritious foods, it will stop craving junk.

4   Your new life-long plan must be something you can live with. There is no point in adopting some strange eating pattern which does not fit in with eating out, and social eating and drinking. The kinds of exercise that you adopt must also be enjoyable to you. Different types of exercise may be easier to live with than a single approach.

5   You must give up any deep-seated fear that carbohydrates are inherently fattening. Any food will make you fat if you eat enough of it. However, carbohydrates contribute fewer kilojoules than any other form of food. The main point to watch is the company your carbohydrates keep. Those which are accompanied by loads of fat will soon pile on the kilos.

6   You must accept your basic body shape. If you are short, you will never look like a tall willowy model. Even the best diet and exercise programme in the world cannot alter your basic bone structure. You can, however, alter the contours of your body by reducing fat and increasing muscle. The more lean muscle tissue you have, the more kilojoules you will be able to eat without gaining fat.

Should you count kilojoules?

The amount of energy that a food can provide is measured in kilojoules (or Calories). Fats contribute 37 kilojoules per gram (or 9 Calories) : they have the highest level. Alcohol has 29 kilojoules per gram (7 Calories), and proteins, at 17 kilojoules per grams (4 Calories), and carbohydrates, at 16 kilojoules per gram (4 Calories), have the lowest levels.

It is tempting to think that the fewer kilojoules you take in, the faster you will lose weight. That is incorrect. Most people lose weight better on 5000 kilojoules (1200 Calories) a day than on 2500 kilojoules. Once the energy level falls below a certain point (generally about 4000 kilojoules per day), the body simply learns to slow down and burn up fewer kilojoules.

145

Kilojoules (or Calories) certainly *do* count. But it is boring to actually count them and, unless you have accurate scales, the kilojoules that you *think* you are having may be quite different from those that you actually are having. As discussed earlier, if the carbohydrate content of the diet is too low, some of the lean muscle tissue will also be lost.

In practice, it is probably better to look at the types of foods you are eating and know which foods you can eat in large quantities (to fill you up) and which need to be consumed only in very small quantities. For example, there is not much point in counting kilojoules in vegetables since they are so low that it hardly matters. However, it could help to know just how many kilojoules foods like chocolates, pastries, cakes and chips really have.

Look for the fibre and carbohydrate

The more fibre a food has, the greater its ability to be satisfying. Rolled oats or wholemeal bread, for example, have no more kilojoules than cornflakes or white bread. But the wholegrain products are much more filling because of their dietary fibre.

Any food which is filling is most unlikely to be fattening since fibre acts as a natural obstacle to overeating. Many people shun filling foods and then spend most of their time thinking about what they will eat. It makes far more sense to have a good meal which satisfies you and then forget about eating for the next few hours.

Foods which are rich in dietary fibre and carbohydrate include:

- wholemeal or wholegrain bread (the former is simply the latter with the grains broken up to produce a smoother texture).
- wholegrain cereals such as oats, wholewheat breakfast biscuits, wheat–based breakfast cereals, brown rice and any grains (such as cracked or whole wheat, rye, barley, millet, buckwheat).
- vegetables of all kinds, including potatoes (*not* chips since they are primarily sources of fat).
- fruits, including the skin where appropriate.
- legumes such as chick peas, lentils, kidney beans, soya and other beans.

These foods might be included in meals such as those that follow:

Breakfast
Rolled oats or a good quality cereal served with low-fat milk
Wholemeal toast
Fruit (if desired)

Lunch
Wholemeal bread sandwich with salad and chicken/turkey/ Weight
    salmon/egg/cottage or low-fat cheese/very lean meat
Fruit or fruit salad

or Large salad with potato
    and/or a wholemeal roll
Fruit

or Baked beans on wholemeal toast
Fruit

or Soup containing beans, barley and vegetables
Wholemeal toast or roll or rye crispbread
Fruit

Dinner
Plenty of vegetables
Pasta or rice or some other grain food served with seafood/
    chicken/turkey/legumes/a small portion of very lean meat
Fruit salad or fresh fruit

Snacks (if needed)
Wholemeal bread, muffins, toast, wholemeal crumpets or whole-
    grain crispbread
Fruit, fresh or dried
Vegetables

How much to eat

Rather than a long list of no-no's, let's take a look at what an overweight person can and should be eating. The following foods represent a minimum. Many people will lose weight quite satisfactorily on larger quantities.

Every day, you should include:

- *At least four slices of bread*, preferably wholemeal. Many men and women who exercise a lot should aim for five to six slices.
- *Lots of vegetables*: any type, except those cooked in fat or oil or with added extra fat in the form of butter, margarine or sour cream.

    There need be no restriction on vegetables but a minimum of three to four types should be eaten each day.

    Vegetables can be raw or cooked in a microwave, steamed, in casseroles or stir-fried (try using concentrated chicken stock instead of oil or fat).

147

Some fresh vegetables should be included, but frozen and canned varieties (preferably the 'no added salt' ranges) will still contribute complex carbohydrate, dietary fibre and most of the vitamins.

- *Two to four pieces of fruit*, any type. Teenagers and those who exercise a lot may need more.
- *Some type of cereal or grain product*: preferably a wholegrain food such as oats, brown rice, cracked wheat, wholemeal pasta, wholewheat breakfast biscuits or a wheat-based breakfast cereal. The serving size will vary from small to large depending on the size and level of physical activity of the individual.
- *One serve of a protein food* such as fish or another seafood, chicken with its fat removed, turkey, very lean red meat (small serve), eggs, cheese (small piece), legumes (dried peas and beans).

  Those who need more than one serve of these foods should make their extra choice seafood, lean poultry or legumes.
- *Some dairy products*: preferably low-fat milk (500ml) or non-fat yoghurt (400g).
- *As little fat as possible*: try to keep butter, margarine, chocolate, oils and cooking fats to a minimum.

The role of exercise

Exercise is important for a healthy body. Those who have plenty of physical activity are much less likely to have a weight problem. Years ago, the daily grind of living entailed a certain amount of physical exercise.

In our age, as soon as any job becomes too strenuous, we have a machine to replace physical effort. We drive, often because we have no time to walk. We have kitchens, houses and offices specially designed to save energy. We spend our leisure time watching television or as spectator sportspeople. We shun most types of physical activity.

It is the lack of physical activity which has caused so many people to be overweight. We do not eat more kilojoules than earlier, thinner generations. We simply exercise less. This alters the balance between what comes into the body from food and what leaves the body for metabolism and physical activity.

Many people have discovered how good they feel when regular exercise becomes a part of their daily routine. Others have tried exercise and have found it tiring. Once you adopt a healthier diet which is high in complex carbohydrate, you will find exercise much easier.

If you look at a chart which tells you how many kilojoules are used for various types of physical activity, you may become disheartened so note how few kilojoules some activities use. However, if performed regularly, the cumulative total of the kilojoules used is significant.

It is also important to note the effect of exercise on metabolism. Hours after exercise, the body will still be using more kilojoules for its metabolism. A brisk 40-minute walk at lunchtime will provide benefits for your body throughout the afternoon. When this added effect of exercise is taken into account, physical activity becomes very valuable in controlling weight.

If you have not exercised much for some years, you may find a temporary increase in weight when you begin an exercise programme. This occurs because the muscle that you are developing weighs more than the fat that it is replacing. It is therefore important not to become discouraged if the scales show a rise of a kilogram or two in the initial weeks of an exercise programme. After several weeks, fat losses will continue to increase and the total weight will drop.

Once you have exercised enough to build up more lean muscle tissue, your need for kilojoules will increase. Exercise, even without dietary change, can thus bring about weight loss. The best results for permanent weight loss, however, come from an exercise programme coupled with changes in eating habits.

If possible, try to fit in 30 to 40 minutes of exercise five times a week. This will not only help you to slim but will increase your cardiovascular fitness, keeping blood fat levels low and decreasing your chances of heart disease.

Giving up smoking

Many people give up smoking and do not gain a gram. Others find that as soon as they stop smoking, the kilos come thick and fast. The fear of weight gain is sufficient to prevent some women from giving up smoking while others foolishly begin to smoke in order to control their weight.

There is no doubt that it is more damaging to smoke than it is to gain weight. But that is not enough to comfort those for whom the dangers of smoking and future health problems pale into insignificance beside the more immediate threat of putting on weight.

If you understand why weight gain so often occurs after you stop smoking, you can give up cigarettes without gaining weight. If you take a total turn for a healthier lifestyle, you can even stop smoking and lose weight. First, let us look at the reasons why weight gain dogs those who give up smoking and how to deal with these.

149

Problem	How to cope
1 Once you stop smoking, your appreciation of the flavours of foods usually increases. Everything tastes so good that you find yourself wolfing down more and more.	Make sure that everything you eat is of top quality. Ask yourself if foods are worth the kilojoules before eating them. With your heightened sense of awareness of flavour and taste, you can begin to appreciate that the enjoyment of food lies in selecting superb–tasting items rather than stuffing yourself with anything.
2 Smoking provides oral gratification. So does eating. Many people simply swap one form for another and eat every time they would previously have had a cigarette.	If you cannot resist the urge to have something in your mouth, try sugarless chewing gum — at least in private.
3 Smoking gives you something to do. So does eating. Many people find a need to mask their slight discomfort at sitting down doing nothing by occupying their hands, either with a cigarette or a drink or with some food.	Find something else to do with your hands. Try worry beads or knitting or crochet, or hold a book. If these are not appropriate to the occasion, set yourself small goals by waiting a certain time before seeking food. As you gain more self-confidence, you can extend the time. Alternatively, try sipping a glass of water, or mineral water or tea.
4 A cigarette often signifies the end of a meal. Without this cue, many people simply go on eating.	Finish a meal with a piece of fresh fruit. For example, you could adopt a habit of eating a few slices of apple after each meal. Or you can avoid having serving dishes on the table for a while. If making yourself a meal or snack, put everything away before you sit down to eat.

150

Problem	How to cope
5 Smoking increases the number of kilojoules your body burns up each day. Everybody is different and there are variations in metabolism between people. In general, however, studies have shown that smoking does use up some kilojoules.	You can also increase the number of kilojoules your body uses by exercising. For many people, more kilojoules will also be used if meals are divided into a series of small snacks throughout the day instead of three regular meals. This also has the advantage of giving more eating occasions.

Ex-smokers' eating plan

This eating plan shows how you can turn your day's foods into a series of healthy snacks which can help to avoid weight gain when you quit smoking.

Breakfast

Do not skip this meal. It has been shown that the metabolism for the entire day is reduced if breakfast is skipped. Choose one of the following and add a cup of tea or coffee and/or a glass of water.

1 Wholewheat breakfast biscuits with low-fat milk.
Wholegrain muffin or wholemeal toast with low-kilojoule jam or Vegemite.

2 Poached or boiled egg on wholemeal toast.
Small piece of fresh fruit.

3 Carton of non-fat yoghurt mixed with one to two pieces of fresh fruit.

4 Grilled mushrooms and tomato.
Wholemeal toast with low-fat cheese.

5 Porridge with wheatgerm and one level teaspoon of brown sugar with low-fat milk.
Wholemeal toast with low-kilojoule jam.

The quantity of toast will depend on the individual. Generally, one slice for women, two for men and more for those who exercise a lot.

During the morning

Choose one or two of the following healthy snacks:

2 whole-rye crispbread with low-kilojoule jam
3 wholegrain crackerbread with ricotta cheese and tomato
2 fresh or dried figs
small packet of sultanas
1 punnet of strawberries
small tub of coleslaw (preferably homemade with low-kilojoule
   dressing)
small can of baked beans
small piece of fresh coconut (about 15g)
small serve of fresh fruit salad
1 piece of fresh fruit, any type except grapes (it is too easy to eat too
   many)
½ cup of buttermilk mixed with ½ cup of orange juice (a refreshingly
   tangy drink)
1 cup of soup, preferably homemade
6 prunes
8–10 pieces of dried apple (their tartness is great when your mouth
   feels awful)
1 hard-boiled egg and some carrot and celery sticks
1 slice of bread with tomato, cucumber, alfalfa or any other salad
   vegetable
low-fat milkshake (blend ¾ cup of skim milk with low-kilojoule
   topping or some instant coffee and icecubes)

Lunch

Choose one of the following:

1   A wholemeal sandwich with salad and either turkey, lean
    chicken, salmon, tuna, cottage cheese or a small slice of very
    lean meat (skip the butter or margarine, and avoid mayon-
    naise).
2   A large salad (use a low-kilojoule dressing) with some rye or
    wholemeal bread or crispbread.
3   One cup of vegetable soup (for example, pumpkin or tomato)
    with wholegrain bread.
4   Half of a small avocado with salad and wholegrain crispbread.
5   Wholemeal pita bread stuffed with salad and hummous or
    felafel (chick pea patties).
6   Large plate of steamed vegetables sprinkled with sesame
    seeds, and some wholegrain bread.

If you are small or fairly sedentary, choose one slice of wholegrain
bread. If you are large and/or very active, choose two or more.

During the afternoon

You may have one or two snacks from the list given for the morning. If you are not hungry, skip snacks.

Dinner

This should be a meal with plenty of vegetables (no added butter or oil or other fat). Add some fish or another seafood, some chicken breast, turkey fillet, new-fashioned pork or veal or legumes. If having red meat, keep to a small piece (about 100 grams) and make sure that it is very lean.

Potato, pasta or rice can be added in a quantity to suit the individual. As before, large and/or active people need larger serves.

Fish and other foods can be cooked by grilling, microwaving, making into a casserole (use a pan liner to brown foods where appropriate), or wrapping them in foil and baking or barbecueing.

After-dinner snack

If hungry, choose one of the following:

- cup of hot skim milk
- 1 cup fresh fruit salad
- bowl of strawberries or other berries
- low-kilojoule jelly
- ¼ rockmelon or honeydew melon sprinkled with 1 teaspoon of concentrated orange juice
- ½ cup of non-fat yoghurt with fresh fruit
- 1 cup of freshly popped corn (try using the microwave, no added butter is needed)
- ½ muffin with low-kilojoule jam
- 1 slice raisin toast with a small scrape of butter
- 2 small water crackers with a sliver of cheese
- 8 olives

What about gaining weight?

It is hard for overweight people to accept, but it can be more difficult for a chronically thin person to gain weight than for the overweight to lose it.

If you are thin, you should first of all consider if any of the following apply:

- You are a smoker.
- You eat very little over a 24-hour period.

153

- You skip meals when you're involved in work or you simply forget to eat.
- You are a fussy eater.
- You exercise a great deal.
- You have very little physical activity.

If none of these apply, and you regularly eat as much as those around you, it may be that you have a body which will be permanently thin. Exercise can help build up muscle tissue and this will certainly help you to look heavier and in better shape.

Exercise is essential for the proper functioning of the appetite-control mechanism. Occasionally, however, people spend so much time exercising that they will not have enough time to eat sufficient food to provide energy for the exercise. Such people are usually lean, but have plenty of muscle development. Eating a little more and/or exercising a little less may help a little more fat to take up residence.

On the other hand, some people who spend their entire lives in sedentary pursuits may not generate sufficient appetite to eat enough. Increasing exercise can help normalise such people's eating habits.

If you don't seem to be able to gain weight, and you are having sufficient exercise, and don't smoke and eat well, you may need to console yourself that your lack of body fat will at least increase your chances of a long life.

12

Eating for peak performance in sport

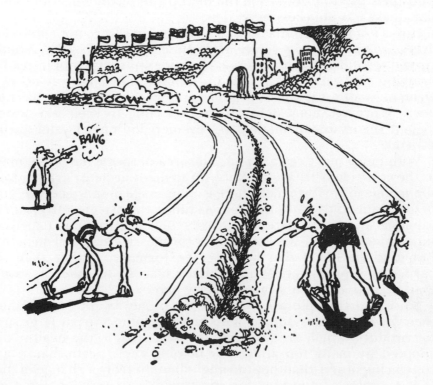

THE history of sport and fitness is riddled with myths and legends. It all began when a fellow named Charmis, of Sparta, reputedly dosed himself with dried figs and then won the 200–yard race in record time in the Olympic Games of 668 BC. Whether it was the natural sugar in the figs, or their well-known laxative effect which got him to the finishing line so fast is not clear. But this gentleman started a long line of spurious connections between food and fitness.

Many sportsmen and women have adopted very healthy diets and are valuable role models for young athletes. Some of the nutrition practices of well-known sportspeople, however, are totally ineffective. Many follow fads and some take expensive supplements which are useless or even hazardous for future health. Footballers, for example, were once urged to eat more protein and they would boast about the size of the steaks they ate before the game (and the amount of beer they drank afterwards). Unfortunately, studies of footballers later in life showed that they had a reduced life expectancy, presumably due to all the fat they inadvertently took in with their protein. And even the high-protein content of the king-size steaks was unnecessary.

It was not long ago that most sporting teams were not allowed to drink water before a game. Half–time was marked by mouths curved around orange quarters as the juice was sucked out instead of drinking the water which the dry mouths indicated was needed. Drinking water was said to produce cramps, an idea which has now been disproved. Some football coaches cling to their old 'water-logged' theory and maintain that 'real men don't need water during a match'.

With much more research into the area of sports nutrition, many of the crazy ideas are going. But with so many athletes striving for a slight edge in performance, there is an upsurge in sportspeople's use of supplements of spurious value. At times, the placebo effect can be valuable and an athlete who really believes that an expensive supplement will provide extra power for muscles may well do better. But it is the belief that improves performance rather than the particular supplement. Many athletes succeed in spite of, rather than because of, their strange dietary habits.

Since sportspeople are regarded so highly by the community, their use of worthless supplements may lead others to pay large sums for products which are fakes. By the same token, the healthy diet adopted by many top athletes is helping their performance and convincing others that they too might benefit from a change of diet. It is therefore important for sportspeople to pick up the right nutrition messages.

The need for fuel

No diet, however good, can improve fitness or sporting ability, by itself. But there is no doubt that a poor diet can ruin one's chances of achieving peak performance.

Muscle cells need fuel. During exercise, you use up about 20 times more energy than when you are sedentary. In theory, all body cells can derive energy from carbohydrates, fats and, if needed, from proteins. Vitamins do not provide energy, although both minerals and vitamins are important in the enzyme systems which control the body's chemistry.

Sprinting, or any short intense muscular action, requires the muscles cells to produce energy in the absence of oxygen. Such activities are known as anaerobic and they cannot be sustained for more than a minute or two. The only fuel which can be used for anaerobic activity is the carbohydrate stored in the muscles as glycogen.

With cycling, distance running, swimming or even walking, oxygen has time to enter the muscle cell and produce a much more efficient aerobic supply of energy. The major fuel for aerobic activity starts off being carbohydrate (again in the form of glycogen), but as the action continues more fatty acids (from fat stores) are used as fuel.

The role of carbohydrates

Carbohydrates are the body's preferred source of energy. They are broken down during digestion and provide glucose. The body can either use glucose 'straight' as a source of energy or convert it to glycogen which is stored in the liver and muscles. If the glycogen stores are full, any excess glucose is converted to body fat.

Glycogen stored in the liver is used mainly to replenish the level of glucose in the blood. A few hours after eating, the blood sugar level will fall slightly. This stimulates a feeling of hunger, telling you that you need something to eat. If you do not eat when you feel hunger pangs, after a few minutes the feeling subsides. The body realises that no food is forthcoming and converts some of the glycogen in the liver into glucose to replenish the blood supply. Once this is used up, another hunger signal goes out. Hopefully, this time you will be able to eat. If not, some more liver glycogen will be used. Once the liver glycogen is used up, if you still do not eat, some of the body's lean tissue will be broken down to provide blood glucose. Fat cannot be changed into glucose.

The glycogen in muscles is for the muscles to use. Very little of this glycogen can be converted into blood sugar because the 157 necessary enzyme to catalyse the reaction is not present in the muscles. The higher the levels of glycogen in the muscles, the longer they can work before fatigue sets in. Marathon runners, triathletes and others who take part in endurance activities therefore try to maximise their muscle glycogen stores. Once the glycogen stores are exhausted, the well-known runner's 'wall' is reached.

What about sugar?

It might appear that the ideal way to replenish blood glucose levels and glycogen supplies would be to eat sugar. While sugar can certainly provide glucose for the blood, it is not the ideal source. Sugar has absolutely no minerals, vitamins or dietary fibre. It enters the bloodstream quickly and that is not ideal as the body must produce more insulin to remove it. Some people produce too much insulin after eating sugar and this causes their blood sugar levels to *fall*. If such a person then begins to exercise, there may be a further drop in blood sugar levels and a loss of performance.

There is no need for athletes to avoid all sugar. But for peak performance, most of the carbohydrate in an athlete's diet should come from sources such as breads, cereals and grain foods (for example, pasta), vegetables and fruits. These foods also supply the vitamins and minerals needed for the body to use the carbohydrates. Small quantities of sugar will not do any harm, as long as the sweet foods chosen are not also high in fat or used in place of other more nutritious foods.

It is unwise to take sugar or glucose, either in food or in a drink, within an hour before an athletic event. Sugar in the stomach causes water to be transferred from other tissues into the stomach and may cause cramps, nausea and diarrhoea.

Once a long endurance event is under way, sugar can be used if plenty of water is also available. After exercise begins, the problem of an oversupply of insulin does not occur since the exercise itself controls the flow of insulin. For events lasting more than a few hours, when some type of food must be eaten, sweet foods or drinks can be useful.

The role of fat

Body fat is a potential source of fuel for exercise. Most people have sufficient body fat to provide fatty acids for fuel for days of continuous physical activity.

The longer exercise lasts, the more fat is used as a source of fuel. It is as if the body knows that it must make its glycogen stores last as long as possible and so switches to the much more abundant fat supply. Highly trained athletes have a much greater ability to use fat as the source of energy for endurance events.

Fatty acids come from the breakdown of body fat or from the fats in foods. Most people have ample supplies of body fat and there is no point in loading the body with heaps of fatty foods. In fact, a high-fat diet tends to produce clogged arteries which impede the flow of blood to the heart and thus reduce capacity for exercise. In practice, a low-fat/high-carbohydrate diet produces the best performance for both health and physical activity.

The role of protein

Protein can be used as a source of energy during exercise, but it contributes a much smaller share of energy than either carbohydrates or fats. The major use for protein is in the repair of muscle cells. It is also required in larger quantities during training and muscular development.

The quantity of glycogen available also influences the amount of protein needed. Once glycogen stores are depleted, more protein is broken down in the body. In endurance events, there is thus a larger loss of protein. The highest requirement for protein among athletes occurs in those who train for endurance events. After 60 to 70 minutes of activity, the rate of protein breakdown increases significantly.

Those involved in body building also need more protein during the phase of building up muscle mass. However, the quantity of extra protein needed is only a fraction of the huge amount often consumed by body builders.

Anyone who is physically active needs more protein than those with a more sedentary lifestyle. This does not mean that footballers who devoured huge steaks were right after all. Nor does it mean that athletes need protein supplements. The typical Western diet is so high in protein that most people are already consuming more than enough for any degree of muscle development or athletic pursuit. The possible exception may occur in some athletes who eat a very narrow range of foods or in strict vegetarians who shun all animal products. However, protein deficiency is extremely rare.

In general, one gram a day of protein for every kilogram of body weight will be more than adequate for most people. Endurance athletes and those involved in body building will usually find this quantity sufficient. Some researchers have recently recommended that these athletes should aim for 1.3 to 1.6 grams of protein per kilogram of body weight. For the average 70–kilogram man, this would mean eating 90 to 110 grams of protein per day. Typical protein intakes for men in Western countries are greater than this so most athletes would already be taking in more than enough protein.

Protein supplements

Studies which have looked for any possible benefits from protein supplements have found none. In spite of their popularity, protein supplements are rarely needed. They can, however, be useful for athletes who feel too nervous before an event to be able to chew foods.

Before paying high prices for protein supplements, take a look at their list of ingredients. Most are based on milk powder, usually skim but occasionally full cream. A few have added soya bean protein which is a reasonable source of protein but in no way superior to other proteins. Most have added sugar and vitamins which can present an excess to an athlete's body.

Skim milk powder is very cheap; most protein supplements are expensive. If you feel that you must have a protein supplement, you can easily and cheaply mix up some skim milk powder with some sugar and flavouring and achieve much the same supplement for about one tenth of the price.

Amino acid supplements

There is a current vogue for amino acid supplements, especially for those involved in some sporting activities or weight training. Amino acids are the materials from which proteins are made.

Ever since steroids were outlawed, athletes have been looking for some way to stimulate growth hormone to produce greater muscle development. One particular amino acid, arginine, is used to test the adequacy of growth hormone in very short children suspected of having a deficiency of this hormone. Arginine is perfused into a vein and its rate of uptake into growth hormone is measured to see if the child is producing a normal quantity of the hormone.

The connection between growth hormone and arginine has been extrapolated to imply that extra arginine will increase production of growth hormone in normal people. Studies have shown a very slight increase in growth hormone after large doses of arginine, but the increase is small and lasts for a very short space of time. The practical effect is nil.

On this spurious basis, sales of arginine, ornithine and other amino acids have been soaring. An examination of the quantities of amino acids present in some supplements showed that a month's supply contained roughly the amino acids found naturally in two eggs! If you are tempted to pay for expensive amino acid supplements, compare the costs with that of two eggs! Amino acids are not 'fat burners', as claimed.

Vitamins

Many people believe that athletes need extra quantities of vitamins. The greatest disciples of this school of thought are those who sell vitamins! Athletes respond by paying large sums for a range of vitamin supplements.

The body's need for some vitamins such as the B-complex does increase with the demands of athletic training. But the higher requirements are only in line with the greater need for kilojoules with more physical activity. Athletes eat more food than their less athletic peers and this extra food can easily provide the extra vitamins required.

The chances of athletes becoming vitamin deficient are no greater than in the general population and very few vitamin deficiencies occur in Western countries. The widespread habit of athletes taking vitamins is of little benefit.

Studies have been carried out to test performance of athletes taking particular vitamins. With vitamin C, there have been ten good, well-controlled studies which have shown no effect of taking supplements. One study which did conclude that some endurance athletes require extra quantities of vitamin C found that the amount could easily be supplied by a normal diet which included fruits and vegetables.

There is concern that some athletes may impair their performance by taking mega-doses of particular vitamins. As noted in chapter 10, too much B_6 can damage the nerve endings in fingers and toes. Large doses of B_6 can also increase the rate at which protein in lean tissue is broken down and hasten the rate at which muscle glycogen is used. It is therefore quite undesirable for athletes to take large doses of this vitamin.

Large doses of niacin (another of the B-complex vitamins) should also be avoided. Excess niacin may inhibit the use of fat as a source of energy. This would be a disadvantage for endurance athletes who rely on the oxidation of free fatty acids for some of their energy.

Vitamins A, thiamin (B_1), riboflavin (B_2), B_{12}, C, D and E have been shown to have no effect in improving athletic performance. Yet there are football players and other sportspeople who line up each week for their shot of B_{12} before a game, believing that it will boost their performance.

The belief in vitamins may well improve performance. But it is important to understand that it is only the belief, not the specific vitamin, which has an effect. The best way to obtain vitamins is from foods. Contrary to claims of some people marketing supplements, foods in Western countries contain plenty of vitamins. And the recommended carbohydrate foods (fruits, vegetables, wholemeal bread, wholegrain cereals and legumes) are especially rich in vitamins.

161

Non-vitamins

There are substances whose virtues are extolled for athletes. They are not officially classified as vitamins, but are sometimes given the title in an effort to bestow biochemical respectability on them. Most are sold at exorbitant prices, the rationale being that anything so expensive must be good. Some are available only on the 'black market', thereby increasing their psychological value.

Vitamin F (or linolenic acid): This polyunsaturated fatty acid is indeed essential, but it does not function as a vitamin. It is found in fish and other seafoods and in linseeds and is related to the omega–3 fatty acids discussed in chapter 2. It is used by the body to make substances called prostaglandins which regulate the membranes around cells. Those with high levels of blood fats may benefit from linolenic acid, but it has no special virtues for athletes.

Vitamin B–T (or carnitine): This substance is important in allowing muscle cells to use fats for fuel. Carnitine is made within the body as required and, as yet, there is no evidence that it has value as a supplement to athletes.

Vitamin P (or bioflavenoids): This group of substances occurs in fruits and vegetables and helps to protect vitamin C from being destroyed by oxygen in the atmosphere. Bioflavenoids also contribute some of the colour to various fruits and are especially rich in citrus fruits. There is no reason why athletes need extra quantities of bioflavenoids: they are well supplied by fruits and vegetables.

Vitamin B_{13} (or orotic acid — the 'o' is not a misprint!): This substance is found in whey (which separates from milk in the making of cheese). It is involved in making both DNA and RNA in the body and is sometimes sold to athletes in the belief that it will increase the ability to produce energy in muscles. In fact, there is no evidence that orotic acid acts as a vitamin and, at present, there is no justification for using expensive supplements of it.

Vitamin B_{15} (or pangamic acid): This substance can be extracted from apricot kernels and is claimed to prevent everything from heart disease, diabetes, schizophrenia, allergies, alcoholism and cancer. None of these claims has ever been substantiated. Most studies have found it to have no effects of benefit to athletes. Since there is some evidence that pangamic acid may be a cancer-causing agent, it should be avoided.

Vitamin B_{17} (or amygdalin, or laetrile): Also extracted from apricot kernels and claimed to cure cancer, this substance is banned since it is a source of cyanide. However, it is sometimes available for a price. There have been deaths from its use and it too should be avoided.

Apricot kernels have no benefits for athletes and eating just 25 of them can be hazardous.

Other supplements

Royal jelly is often taken by athletes in the hope that it will confer some of the benefits it obviously has for the queen bee. There is no evidence that it will do any good, apart from the belief that it might. It is rich in pantothenic acid (one of the B–complex vitamins), but this vitamin is unlikely to be in short supply in our bodies.

Bee pollen is widely used by athletes who claim that it helps their performance. Pollen contains amino acids, but has no specific properties to benefit humans. Again, it is probably the belief in it which is responsible for some satisfied users.

Minerals and trace elements

Unlike vitamins, there are some minerals which may need attention in an athlete's diet.

Iron: As mentioned in chapter 9, some women, including athletes, lack iron. Since iron is involved in carrying oxygen in the blood, it is obviously important to sports performance. To remedy an iron deficiency it may be advisable to use iron tablets. These should also contain vitamin C to assist in the absorption of the iron. If iron tablets cause constipation, try a change of tablet. Ferrous fumarate may cause less upset to the intestine than ferrous sulphate. Iron-rich foods include kidney, liver, oysters, lean red meat, chicken, turkey, dried fruits, wholemeal bread, breakfast cereals, rolled oats, eggs, lentils, broccoli and other green vegetables (see chapter 9 for further details).

Calcium: Female athletes who have very low levels of body fat may find that their hormonal levels change and periods cease. If this happens, there is also a danger that the amount of calcium being lost from the bones will increase rapidly. Studies of female athletes have indicated that such very lean women run a greatly increased risk of osteoporosis (see chapter 9). The solution to this problem may be unpalatable to some elite athletes since it involves allowing body fat levels to increase to the point where menstruation returns. Taking extra calcium (from foods or supplements) will be insufficient to correct the effects of the hormonal changes.

Sodium, potassium, chloride and magnesium: Each of these minerals is lost in sweat to some extent, with lower losses in trained athletes. They are all easily replaced from the normal diet and there is generally no need for them to be given as supplements or in sports drinks.

Taking salt tablets for extra sodium can be dangerous and is not advisable. Salt losses in sweat are best replaced from the salt present in foods (naturally present in meat, milk and eggs and added to breads, cereals and cheeses). Taking salt tablets after exercise will draw fluid into the intestine and can cause cramps, nausea and dizziness.

Drinks

Nearly two-thirds of a lean body is water. Heavy exercise can cause water losses of up to a litre per hour. This must be replaced to prevent the dehydration which will decrease the ability of the muscles to use energy. Loss of water will prevent peak performance.

During exercise, far more water than salt is lost from the body. After this fluid loss, the salt remaining in the body actually becomes more concentrated. Adding further salt adds insult to injury. It is essential to replace lost water before replacing lost salt.

The ideal fluid to replace losses is plain water. Sports drinks are popular, but they are not essential. Some are not even well designed and contain far too much sodium and potassium. If you want to use such products, make sure that you select one with low levels of electrolytes. The maximum recommended sodium level is 10 meq (230 mg/L); potassium should not exceed 5 meq (195 mg/L).

With endurance events, water needs to be replaced during the event. If the water is in the form of a glucose solution, it will not empty from the stomach as quickly as plain water. Studies have shown that fifteen minutes after drinking 400 millilitres of cold water, 60 to 70 per cent of the water will have emptied from the stomach into the small intestine. When the same volume of water contains 10 per cent glucose (the same quantity found in juices, soft drinks and some sports drinks), less than 5 per cent will have left the stomach after fifteen minutes. Added glucose or sugar can form 2 to 3 per cent of the contents of a drink (this is about one quarter of the level in fruit juices, soft drinks and many sports drinks).

Most of us are accustomed to drinking when we are thirsty. After a heavy loss of fluid, it can take up to 48 hours for the thirst mechanism to tell you to drink enough to replace the losses. Those who train hard regularly must therefore drink more than they think they need. A good way to tell how much you need to drink is to weigh yourself before and after a training session. The difference in weight represents the amount of fluid lost. This should be replaced before the next training session.

Many athletes still believe that drinking water before exercise will cause cramps. It won't. Dehydration during exercise can be forestalled by taking about 500 millilitres of water ten to fifteen minutes beforehand. With any endurance event, try to drink plenty of water for a day or two beforehand.

After physical activity, it is important to replace water losses before having alcohol or salt. The exercise will have created a state of partial dehydration; alcohol or salt will enhance it. So have plenty of water before starting on beer.

Glucose polymer drinks

These new products contain 5 per cent glucose in a form which empties from the stomach as fast as plain water. Some athletes find them useful in long term events or on days when there are multiple events.

Tea and coffee

Both tea and coffee contain caffeine. Average-strength tea has about half the caffeine content of coffee. Strong brewed coffee has about twice the caffeine of regular coffee. Chocolate and cola drinks also contain caffeine.

Caffeine does not accumulate in the body, but acts as a diuretic and encourages water loss from the kidneys. In large doses, caffeine stimulates the central nervous system and may increase the heart rate. Whether you are an athlete or not, it is unwise to drink more than three to five cups of coffee a day.

Caffeine can increase the oxidation of free fatty acids, thus sparing glycogen, and some athletes drink large quantities of flat cola beverages or coffee in an attempt to shift the production of energy onto fat and make muscle glycogen last longer. However, the extra caffeine has a diuretic effect and the loss of fluid may have more disadvantages than the prospect of sparing a little glycogen.

The energy requirements for various types of activity

Different types of physical activity use up varying amounts of energy. In general, however, the energy requirement is related to the size of the person (it takes more energy to move a large body) and to the length of time devoted to the activity. Details of the energy required for various activities are given below.

Walking

You can calculate the amount of energy you use for walking from a well-established formula.

Energy used (kJ) = distance travelled (km) × body weight (kg) × 4.2   165

A 60–kilogram person walking five kilometres would therefore use 1260 kilojoules (300 Calories). An 80–kilogram person walking the same distance would use 1680 kilojoules (400 Calories). Thus the heavier the body, the greater the energy needed to move it. For this reason, those who are overweight and take up walking will find that they are likely to lose weight. As explained earlier, exercise also increases the body's rate of burning up energy for its metabolic processes for some hours after the exercise ceases.

Running

The energy cost of running varies according to the weight of the person and the speed of the run. If you run on sand, almost twice as much energy is needed. In general, running (but not sprinting) uses up a similar amount of energy to walking for a given distance. Running five kilometres thus burns as many kilojoules as walking the same distance. Running takes less time, but walking has the advantage of being unlikely to cause any injury.

Cycling

The energy cost of cycling depends on the bike, the weight of the cyclist and whether it occurs on hills, flat ground or on an exercise bike.

A 70–kilogram person can use anything from 1000 to 2500 kilojoules per hour with road cycling. These figures would be altered by about 14 per cent for each 10 kilograms' difference in body weight of the cyclist.

With an exercise bicycle, it is easier to work out the energy requirements, according to the formula:

$$\text{Energy used (kJ/min)} = \frac{\text{workload (Watts)} \times 12.24 + 300}{47.6}$$

Pedalling at a workload of 100 Watts would use up 32 kJ (7.5 Calories) per minute.

Squash

Again, the level of energy uses will vary according to how fast the game is played. A 70–kilogram person would use up anything from 1200 to 2100 kJ (285 to 500 Calories) in a 30-minute game. For lighter or heavier body weights, this figure would be reduced or increased by about 14 per cent.

Tennis

Social tennis generally uses much less energy than the game played at a competitive level. Our 70–kilogram person enjoying a social game would use up around 750 kJ (180 Calories) in 30 minutes. A person of the same weight playing competition tennis would use up twice as much.

Swimming

For swimming to use up significant amounts of energy and to provide cardiovascular fitness, it needs to be done continuously over a period of 30 minutes or so. The energy used will depend on the proficiency of the swimmer, but will not change much for different weight people since the water bears the body weight. At any easy pace, swimming freestyle uses up about twice as much energy as breaststroke. At higher levels of pace, there is little difference in energy expenditure for different strokes.

A good hard 30 minutes of swimming will use up 1900 to 2200 kJ (450 to 525 Calories). Easy swimming uses up about one third of this amount.

Aerobics

There is a wide variation in the amount of energy used during aerobic dancing. A 60–kilogram person will generally expend somewhere between 800 and 1200 kJ (190 to 290 Calories) per session. For every extra 10 kilograms of body weight, these figures will be increased by about 14 per cent.

Football

During a game of football, a player may run anywhere between 6 and 20 kilometres. This would correspond to 2000 to 6700 kJ (480 to 1600 Calories) of energy used by an 80–kilogram player. The exact energy use will depend on the code of football and the position being played.

Cricket

A game of cricket can provide a variety of different levels of energy use. Some players use little energy. A bowler (with a weight of 70 kilograms) might use 1600 kJ (380 Calories) per hour. A reasonably active batsman would expend around the same amount of energy.

Endurance events

The limiting factor for endurance events is the muscles' stores of glycogen. The speed with which glycogen is used will depend on the intensity of the effort, the length of time of the event and the amount of glycogen stored in the muscles. Both the amount of glycogen stored in the muscles and the time to exhaustion are influenced by diet.

167

During any endurance event, the chief fuels for the muscles are glycogen stores in the muscles and in the liver, and some fatty acids. Once the muscle glycogen is exhausted, muscle fatigue occurs. The major goal for such events is therefore to minimise the rate of use of glycogen. With increased training, the body is able to make greater use of fats as an energy source. This does not mean that the diet should contain more fat, since even a lean athlete has far greater stores of fat than of glycogen. However, it does emphasise the need for adequate training for any long-term event.

Once an endurance event is under way, foods containing sugar can be included. These will not influence the muscle glycogen, but will help to keep the blood sugar level normal. Sugar is not a suitable food just before an event. However, once exercise begins, there is a reduction in the concentration of insulin in the blood and small quantities of sweet foods are well tolerated. Recent studies have shown that eating carbohydrate of any type during prolonged exercise delays muscle fatigue.

The most important consideration in endurance events is water. Small quantities of sodium, potassium and magnesium can be added to drinking water, along with 2 to 3 per cent glucose. During an event lasting a few hours, most competitors will be most comfortable taking only liquids. For longer events, some solid foods may also be desirable. These should always be taken in small quantities and with sufficient water to dilute the stomach contents so that water is not taken from the tissues. Suitable foods include diluted fructose, glucose or sugar-sweetened drinks, diluted fruit juices, fresh or dried fruits, or cakes containing bananas or other fruits. Some people enjoy potatoes or small serves of pasta, and cyclists and skiers find sandwiches or bread rolls appropriate during a long-term event. Fatty foods are totally unsuitable as they will remain in the stomach for too long. High-protein foods are also unsuitable as they do not provide readily available fuel.

Carbohydrate loading

The practice of carbohydrate loading was recommended for some years when it was found that athletes could increase glycogen stores by manipulating their diet and training sessions for a week or so beforehand. Using carbohydrate loading, it was possible to double glycogen stores. Since glycogen is stored in the muscles with water, it follows that as the increased store of glycogen is used, the extra water also becomes available.

The early method of carbohydrate loading involved first depriving the muscles of glycogen by eating no carbohydrates while exercising as much as possible. This was followed by a period of rest combined with eating large amounts of carbohydrate. Many athletes came to hate the technique since the initial depletion phase made them feel extremely tired and the extra fluid which accumulated with the glycogen load made them feel uncomfortably bloated. There were also some cases of changes in heart rhythm during the carbohydrate depletion phase.

These days, it is generally considered that a high-complex carbohydrate diet followed all the time achieves most of the benefits of the old-style carbohydrate loading. Training itself increases the amount of glycogen stored in muscles and a continual supply of carbohydrate will increase these stores further. This involves eating much more carbohydrate than is usual. To make room for it, less fat should be eaten.

If desired, a modified carbohydrate loading technique can be followed by eating moderate quantities of carbohydrate about a week before an event and cutting back on training. This is followed by a further reduction in training and a diet which is extremely high in carbohydrate.

For short-term events, such as sprints or weight lifting, carbohydrate loading is not advisable because of the retention of extra fluid in the muscles. It is totally unnecessary for sports such as football or other activities of less than two hours' duration.

A typical high-carbohydrate menu

Breakfast
Fruit juice
Large serve of wholegrain cereal with dried fruits and banana
Low-fat milk
Wholemeal toast or muffins or crumpets with jam or honey
If a hot dish is required, baked beans are ideal

Morning snack
Bread or toast or fruit loaf or fruit

Lunch
Fruit juice
Sandwiches or rolls (preferably using wholemeal bread, little or no butter and a low-fat filling such as salad and turkey or banana or baked beans)
Fruit (fresh and/or dried)

Afternoon snack
Milkshake using low-fat milk and banana
Rye crispbread or fruit bun

169

Dinner
Fruit juice
Large serve of pasta with seafood and vegetables
Bread or roll
Fruit salad

The pre-event meal

The glycogen in your muscles will have accumulated from the
carbohydrates you have eaten for the day or two before any event.
What you eat on the day of an event will not influence these stores
although it will affect your blood sugar level and liver glycogen. By
morning, most of the previous day's liver glycogen will have been
used so the pre-event meal is important to replenish this and to keep
the blood sugar level normal. While muscle glycogen provides the
fuel for exercise, the blood sugar level will control the functioning
of the brain and nervous system. Should the blood sugar level fall,
reaction times could be adversely affected.

The pre-event meal

1   Have it two to three hours before the event. This will allow
     time for the food to be digested, but not so much time that you
     will feel hungry at starting time.
2   Make sure that you drink plenty of liquid, preferably water.
     Diluted fruit juice would also be suitable, but should not be
     used in the hour before the event. Continue to drink water at
     regular intervals until competition begins.
3   Include carbohydrate, preferably in a form with some dietary
     fibre. Suitable foods would include cereals, wholemeal bread,
     muffins, rice, pasta, vegetables such as potato, or fruit.
4   Avoid foods high in fat or protein. The pre-event meal needs
     to have left the stomach by the time of the event and fats and
     protein take a long time to be digested.
5   Eat foods which are familiar and enjoyable. If you know that
     certain foods do not sit comfortably in your stomach, avoid
     them. You should also avoid foods which you know give you
     wind.
6   Avoid large quantities of sugar or glucose. These sugars
     increase the level of blood sugar and cause an increased
     production of insulin. This will cause muscle glycogen to be
     used faster. It is especially important to avoid taking sugar in
     foods or drinks in the hour before any event.

170

A suitable pre-event meal might be:

Wholewheat breakfast biscuits with banana or another fruit
Low-fat milk
Fruit juice
Wholemeal toast or muffins or pancakes (made without fat) with jam
   or honey but very little butter or margarine
If you want something hot, a poached egg or some pasta would be
   suitable

or

Spaghetti, noodles, rice or potatoes with vegetables
Bread
Fruit

Frequent events

For those athletes involved in several events during a day, it can be
difficult to organise eating. It is important to drink plenty of water
(even for swimmers). If you have more than two hours between
events, you could also eat small quantities of foods which contain
carbohydrate. Bananas, fruits, bread or sandwiches, juices, a little
low-fat milk or some crispbread may be useful. Avoid foods
containing fats and too much protein as these take too long to be digested.

The training diet

Essentially, the training diet follows the same principles which have
been espoused throughout this book. The diet should have:

1   Lots of water.
2   Plenty of complex carbohydrate from breads, cereals and
    grains, vegetables and legumes (the exact quantity will
    depend on the individual, but most athletes will need a
    minimum of six to eight slices of bread plus plenty of cereal
    foods and vegetables).
3   Fruit, both fresh and dried (at least three times a day).
4   Either fish, seafood, turkey, chicken, very lean red meat, low-
    fat cheese, eggs (not fried) or a vegetarian alternative such as
    chick peas, tofu (soya bean curd), or some type of dried beans,
    peas or lentils (one serving a day, or more if appropriate).
5   Very little fat of any type (this includes butter, margarine,
    oils, cooking fats, chocolate, pastries, pies, biscuits, cakes and
    rich desserts).

171

6 Some dairy products, preferably low-fat varieties, including 500 millilitres of low-fat milk (those who cannot eat dairy products will need to eat plenty of fish with edible bones, green leafy vegetables, and soya bean products, or use a calcium supplement).

7 As little alcohol as is socially acceptable.

8 Very little added salt (the salt present naturally in foods and added to products such as bread, cereals and cheese will be ample).

9 Not too much sugar (the quantity will depend on the individual, but sweet foods should not crowd out more nutritious foods).

10 Not more than three to five cups of coffee a day. Extra cups of weak tea are fine.

In addition, athletes should not use mega–doses of vitamins and should try to avoid fads.

13

Planning the day's meals
How many meals?

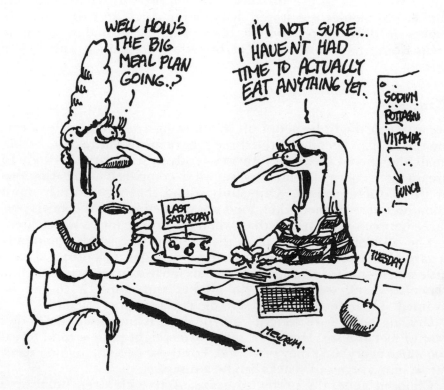

THE idea of eating three meals a day probably developed because it takes four to five hours for an average meal to be digested. If you eat soon after getting up, you are likely to feel hungry by about noon. Lunch removes the hunger pangs for a further five hours or so, until it is time for dinner. Once you fall asleep, the body cuts down the amount of energy it uses, so that you can make it through the night without hunger pangs. By morning, you should be ready to eat again. However, if your dinner is sufficiently large and eaten late, breakfast may have little appeal.

In many countries, the day's main meal is eaten at lunchtime, followed by a siesta to allow the digestive processes to begin their tasks in peace. Once the energy from the food begins to filter through , work is resumed. Such an eating pattern makes far more sense than the common Western practice of eating little breakfast and lunch and ending the day with a large meal. Just when the energy is coming into the body, it is time for bed.

Many overweight people eat very little during the day and make up for it by eating a large dinner and continuing to nibble in front of the television throughout the evening. With such an eating pattern, the body learns to use up very little energy during the day and dinner's kilojoules are stored as body fat. Such an eating pattern makes it difficult to control body weight. It makes sense to redistribute food with more at breakfast and lunch and less at dinner.

'Grazing'

Some people might be better off by adopting a 'grazing' style of eating rather than keeping to the three square meals of the past. Eating small amounts at frequent intervals tends to stimulate the body to use up more energy for metabolism when compared with eating two or three discrete meals. One study found that significantly more kilojoules were burned when food was divided into three meals plus three between-meal snacks than when only three meals were eaten.

The problem with grazing is that most of the foods commonly regarded as snacks tend to be high in fat or sugar, or both, and have little nutritional value. If grazing means more cakes, biscuits, lollies, chocolate bars, soft drinks, doughnuts and chips, it should be avoided. These foods are not suitable replacements for meals.

Grazing helps with weight control since it increases the body's rate of metabolism. However, some overweight people tend to eat too much every time they face food. For these people, turning three meals into a series of snacks can be a disaster.

Children generally prefer to graze. Active children burn up a great deal of energy, but may not have the patience to sit at the table at mealtimes long enough to take in sufficient food to supply their high energy needs. With their high requirements for nutrients for growth and physical activity, children's snacks or 'grazing' foods should feature items such as bread, sandwiches, rolls, muffins, wholewheat breakfast biscuits or other good-quality cereals, wholegrain crispbread, fruit, crisp vegetables, yoghurt, milkshakes (made with low-fat milk and fresh fruit), cheese or eggs.

Many sportspeople also find that grazing is better suited to their lifestyle. Eating small amounts of food often and avoiding a full stomach makes it easier for those who have frequent exercise periods.

BREAKFAST

Breakfast is the most neglected meal of the day, yet it is probably the most important. After an overnight period without food, the body needs to break its fast, replenish liver glycogen levels and provide fuel for the day's activities. Studies have shown that when breakfast is missed, the body's rate of metabolism (that is, the energy used for its basic processes) remains low for the entire day.

Children who have not eaten breakfast suffer a significant drop in concentration levels during the late morning hours while a higher level of industrial accidents occurs in adults who have missed breakfast.

Babies wake in the morning, eager and ready to eat. At some stage between birth and school age, many children give up eating breakfast. Often this change occurs because children stay up late at night and are too tired to get up early enough to have breakfast.

Some people skip breakfast, thinking that the morning rush will carry them through and they will manage to lower their total food intake. Skipping this meal is not a good way to save kilojoules since less energy will be used by the body for the rest of the day. And, without breakfast, high-kilojoule snacks such as doughnuts, biscuits and pastries become very tempting.

What if you cannot eat breakfast?

Some people maintain that the thought of eating breakfast makes them feel sick. If you feel like this about breakfast, you should try getting up a little earlier so that your body has time to adjust to the morning. A short walk (say for ten minutes) may get your body going. Many people find that eating some fresh fruit helps.

You may also find that a breakfast drink will go down more easily than solid food. There are many different delicious and nutritious drinkable breakfasts (see page 178).

175

If you really cannot eat any breakfast, plan to have something to eat as soon as you can. Eating first thing is ideal but eating at eight or nine or even ten o'clock is the next best thing. If you are not at home or in a place where you can prepare food, you will need to take a healthy mid–morning snack with you. This should contain some carbohydrate to replenish the supplies of glycogen in the liver and to prevent the breakdown of lean muscle tissue (see page 58).

Suitable foods to take for a mid-morning snack could include:

- Fruit, either fresh or dried with some yoghurt.
- A sandwich, with whatever filling you please, perhaps banana (sprinkle with lemon juice to prevent browning) or thinly sliced Swiss cheese or turkey ham or light cream cheese and chopped dried apricots or turkey breast with cranberry sauce or chicken.
- Some crispbread or whole breakfast biscuits spread with a little butter and Vegemite or light cream cheese with sliced banana.

Breakfast ideas at home

Breakfast does not need to be cooked. The main requirement is that it contains some carbohydrate, preferably from fruit, breads, cereals, grains or vegetables.

The ideal breakfast includes:

- Fruit.
- Wholegrain cereal with milk (preferably low fat) and/or wholemeal bread or toast or muffins.
- Something to drink (water, low-fat milk, juice, tea or coffee).

Optional extras might be:

- An egg, boiled, poached, coddled, cooked in the microwave (prick the yolk), or scrambled.
- Baked beans or mushrooms or tomatoes or sweet corn.

Suitable wholegrain cereal products include rolled oats (eaten as porridge or raw), wheatgerm (rich in vitamin E), natural muesli (preferably homemade, see recipe in Appendix 1e), wholewheat breakfast biscuits, bran flakes, wheat-based or one of the combination prepared cereals (check that they do not contain too many types of sugar).

Avoid too much butter or margarine on toast or muffins. The sugar in marmalade, honey and jams should not present any

problems when eaten with wholemeal toast or bread. Vegemite is rich in vitamins of the B–complex. It also contains salt, although a thin spread has less salt than the slice of bread with which it is eaten. If you choose peanut butter, use a brand which contains ground-up peanuts, but no salt, sugar or other additives. Peanut butter is rich in niacin (one of the B–complex vitamins) and protein, but also contains fat so it should be used in place of, rather than in addition to, butter or margarine.

An egg is a handy addition to breakfast, especially for those who find cereal and toast does not last much past ten o'clock. Eggs are a good all-round source of nutrients and are not particularly high in fat. However, they do contain ready-made cholesterol so they do not combine well with fatty foods such as bacon or sausages. Eaten without fat, an egg is a healthy food. Bacon and eggs should be eaten rarely.

If you want something unusual for breakfast, that is fine. If pasta or potatoes, rice or ratatouille takes your fancy, there is no reason why you should not have them.

Breakfast for those who need to reduce blood fats

Choose fresh fruit plus rolled oats or a wholegrain breakfast cereal with low-fat milk. Avoid toasted muesli (except for a homemade version as given on page 194) as the commercial varieties are high in fat. Adding a tablespoon or two of oat bran to your cereal can help to reduce blood cholesterol levels.

After your cereal have some wholemeal toast or wholegrain muffins with jam, honey, banana or cottage cheese and tomato. If you want a hot dish, add baked beans or sweet corn or tomatoes or mushrooms or a boiled or poached egg (not more than three times a week). Avoid butter, margarine, cream, bacon and other meats.

Breakfast for those who need to reduce weight

Choose a medium-sized bowl of wholegrain cereal such as rolled oats, wholewheat breakfast biscuits, puffed wheat, bran flakes, any of the wheat-based cereals or one of the better-quality combination cereals (avoid toasted muesli and have only a small serving of any other types of muesli as it is more concentrated). Add low-fat milk, but avoid using sugar.

Wholemeal toast or muffins are suitable, but keep butter or margarine to a minimum (or avoid altogether). Low-kilojoule jams are generally good quality and contain plenty of fruit, but no sugar. Avoid those containing sorbitol, as this has as many kilojoules as sugar. The quantity of toast will depend on the individual. If you are a small person or fairly sedentary, have one slice only. If you are

177

larger and more active, have two or more slices and/or add some
fruit.

If you feel like a hot dish, have a boiled or poached egg, baked
beans or grilled or microwaved tomatoes and/or mushrooms.

Breakfast for those who must avoid salt

Choose rolled oats or homemade muesli or puffed wheat or a cereal
marked 'no added salt'. Add fresh or dried fruit if desired.

Look for wholemeal toast or muffins labelled 'no added salt' or
'low salt' and use butter or margarine with no added salt. Jams and
honey are salt-free, but yeast extracts are not.

If you want a hot dish, have an egg or canned corn, beans or tomatoes with no added salt.

Breakfast for athletes

Choose a regular breakfast with large serves of cereals, fruits, bread,
toast or muffins. The exact quantity will depend on your degree of
physical activity, but you should aim to eat plenty of complex
carbohydrate foods and not too much fat. If you do not want a large
breakfast, at least try to include carbohydrate foods. You should also
remember to drink plenty of water.

Breakfasts you can drink

On those occasions when you have little time for breakfast, you can
whip up a fast and healthy concoction in a blender. Try one of the
following ideas:

- A glass of orange juice with an egg, two tablespoons of skim
  milk powder and a teaspoon of honey.
- A glass of low-fat milk, a banana, half a cup of yoghurt and a
  tablespoon of wheatgerm.
- A small carton of yoghurt and half a cup of strawberries or
  mango or rockmelon or watermelon or any other fruit on
  hand.
- Some melon, mango, papaw, passionfruit (or any combination
  of fruits) with half a carton of natural yoghurt, half a cup of
  milk and a couple of icecubes (choose low-fat yoghurt and milk
  if desired).
- A glass of low-fat milk, a tablespoon of malted milk powder
  and a banana.
- A glass of apple juice with two tablespoons of skim milk
  powder, half an apple (remove core) and a pinch of cinnamon.
- Half a cup of buttermilk with half a cup of orange juice or
  apricot nectar, a slice of rockmelon and two icecubes.

Since these drinkable breakfasts are rather 'light', try to have a slice of wholemeal bread or toast, a sandwich or some wholegrain crispbread during the morning.

LUNCH

By lunchtime, the morning's food will have been used. If you skip lunch, you will first use up some of the liver glycogen stores. After a few hours, these stores will be exhausted and some of your lean muscle tissue wil be broken down to replenish blood sugar levels. To avoid the loss of this lean muscle tissue, you need some lunch.

Sandwiches or bread rolls or pita bread make an easy choice. Choose wholemeal bread, skip the butter or margarine if possible and select healthy fillings.

Suitable fillings include:

- Salad of vegetable and/or potato or coleslaw or tabbouli or Waldorf (apple, celery and walnuts).
- Salad with chicken.
- Salad with turkey breast or turkey ham or turkey salami (all very low in fat).
- Salad with salmon or tuna.
- Salad with egg.
- Salad with very lean meat.
- Salad with cottage cheese or a slice of Swiss cheese.
- Cottage cheese, avocado and alfalfa.
- Cottage cheese with dried fruits and walnuts or pecans.
- Ricotta cheese and banana.
- Peanut butter (no added salt or sugar) with raisins or banana.
- Sliced potato (boiled), apple and cheese .
- Turkey ham and pineapple.
- Baked beans.

Those who are physically active can eat as many sandwiches as their appetite dictates. Those who have a fairly sedentary lifestyle should eat one or two sandwiches.

Other suitable lunch foods include:

- Soup and a wholemeal bread roll.
- Any kind of salad (use a no oil dressing) with crispbread or bread roll.
- Beans on toast.
- Pasta or rice dishes with vegetables (avoid fatty meats and rich sauces).
- Vegetable dishes with wholemeal bread.

179

- Fish or other seafood with potatoes, rice, pasta or bread (avoid fried seafoods).
- Pizza (with a bread dough base rather than a pastry base).

Finish lunch with fruit.

Lunch for those who need to reduce blood fats

Choose a sandwich or roll or pita bread (ask for no butter or margarine) with a filling of salad (without mayonnaise) with chicken or turkey or tuna or salmon or cottage cheese or ricotta or a thin slice of very lean beef. Baked beans, dried fruits, a few walnuts, any type of fruit or vegetable are also suitable.

Soups (made without cream), rice, pasta dishes (without creamy sauces), seafoods (grilled), salads with no oil dressings and any vegetables are also suitable.

If you are eating at a restaurant, you will need to ask for foods to be cooked and served without added fats, oil or cream-based sauces. Grilled fish or other seafoods, turkey breast, pork fillet or a very small lean steak are the best choices. Ask for vegetables to be served without butter and salads without dressing. Eat your bread or roll but skip the butter. If dessert is unavoidable, try to keep to fruit of some kind or choose a sorbet.

If you need a take-away lunch and sandwiches or rolls are not available, Lebanese bread wrapped around tabbouli or felafel is fine, and an occasional slice of pizza will not provide too much fat, as long as it has a bread dough base rather than pastry.

Lunch for those who need to reduce weight

Do not skip lunch. Choose a wholemeal sandwich or roll or pita bread without butter or margarine. Any of the fillings listed on page 179 will be suitable. For most overweight people, one sandwich will be sufficient. If you work hard physically, have a second sandwich or roll with a filling of salad. Add a piece of fruit.

If you are eating in a restaurant, select seafoods (ask for grilled fish without added butter), salads (ask for no dressing), turkey, chicken, pork fillet (without cream sauces) or a small lean grilled steak. You can also order two entrees in place of an entree and a main course. Skip dessert.

Take-away foods are almost all high in kilojoules. A small cheeseburger or a small portion of pizza are the best choices if sandwiches or salads are not available.

Lunch for those who must avoid salt

Choose a sandwich made from low-salt bread or use unsalted crispbread. Suitable fillings include salad vegetables, chicken or turkey, unsalted canned salmon or tuna, egg, jack cheese (it has no added salt), low-salt cottage cheese, lean roast meat (avoid processed meats), any kind of fresh or dried fruit, or unsalted peanut butter.

Other dishes will need to be especially prepared without added salt. If you are eating out, you can generally request a salad without dressing or have some grilled fish or a lean steak with vegetables. In each case, you will need to specifically ask for no salt to be added to your meal. Fast foods are difficult. If unavoidable, have a sandwich or fish or a hamburger and ask for no salt to be added.

Lunch for athletes

Follow the general guidelines, but have larger quantities. Appetite will generally provide a good guide to the quantities needed as long as foods with plenty of dietary fibre are selected. Avoid fatty foods. Athletes are not immune to the effects of fat clogging up arteries.

Eating out at lunchtime

Many restaurants are beginning to cater to those who do not want the afternoon to be a write-off. If possible, look for places that serve foods which are not swimming in fats and where the servings are not gargantuan! If you intend to work in the afternoon, it is socially acceptable these days to drink mineral water in place of wine. For appropriate menu selections, see pp 186–90.

DINNER

Dinner is the meal when most people find time to relax. It is also the meal when most people eat far more food than their bodies need. Healthy eating does not mean that you must lose all the pleasures of the dinner table. Rather than eating huge servings of fat-laden foods, it makes better sense to go for lighter meals with more vegetables, seafoods, chicken or turkey or only small serves of very lean meat.

Most dinner plates feature whatever meat is being served and vegetables are added almost as an afterthought. By changing the order and making vegetables the star performers and meat the accompaniment, you can have a more easily digested and better-balanced meal. Your plate may look as full, but the fat content will be much less.

Foods such as pasta, rice, potatoes, cracked wheat and various types of beans and peas provide valuable complex carbohydrate: these are ideal for those who are physically active.

For vegetables to play a more important role, they need to be well prepared. Cooking vegetables in a saucepan of water and boiling them until they are thoroughly 'dead' is a good way to destroy both

181

the flavour and the vitamins. Try to cook vegetables so that they are still crisp and colourful when served and you will find that they have far more flavour. Cooking vegetables without water in a microwave until they are just tender is ideal. Steaming is almost as good and stir frying is also suitable. Try using about a quarter of a cup of concentrated chicken stock in place of oil. To make chicken stock cover some chicken bones with water, add a few herbs, peppercorns and a bayleaf or two and cook for about an hour. Strain, allow to cool and remove any fat from the top. Use in soups or for stir-fried vegetables.

Salad vegetables come in a far greater range than the ubiquitous lettuce. Look out for some more interesting additions such as raddichio (a purple vegetable with a tangy flavour), cos or mignonette lettuce, curly endive, Belgian endive (also called witlof), watercress, fresh asparagus (available in Spring), red and green capsicum, various sprouts (alfalfa, sunflower, lentil, mung bean), or flavoursome Lebanese cucumbers. Add some snipped fresh herbs such as basil, savoury, Italian parsley, coriander, chives, or thyme. After tossing salad vegetables together, add a healthy dressing made from lemon or lime juice with a little mustard, a small spoonful of honey and some wine or cider vinegar. If you like, use one of the commercial no oil dressings: they have no fat although most are quite salty.

Fish is a healthy addition to a meal. Fresh fish fillets or whole fish can easily be cooked by the following method: Place individual fillets or a whole fish onto a large square of foil. Sprinkle with a little lemon juice. Add a few snipped herbs and vegetables, such as mushrooms or spring onions. Wrap up the parcels and bake in a moderate oven until fish flakes easily with a fork (about 20 minutes for fillets and 40 to 60 minutes for a whole fish).

Fish can also be baked, cooked on the barbeque (using foil as described above), grilled, cooked in the microwave (try wrapping in baking paper), or fried using a pan liner. Try to avoid battered fish as the added fat removes the nutritional virtues of the fish.

Canned tuna and salmon are also good fish choices. Both have a high content of the omega-3 fatty acids described on page 22. Use them in salads, in sauces for pasta or rice, on sandwiches, or in various dishes with vegetables.

Chicken and turkey are low-fat foods, providing that the skin and the underlying layer of fat on the chicken are removed. If you cannot manage to give up chicken skin, at least scrape away any fat under the skin. Chicken breast, turkey fillets and turkey breast are all very low in fat. Turkey ham and turkey salami are also low-fat foods made entirely from lean turkey meat. As a bonus, they have much less salt than their traditional meat-based counterparts.

There is some dispute as to whether chicken or red meat have the most fat. Chicken breast is extremely lean and has *less* fat than meat. Chicken thighs, eaten with their fat intact have more fat than a small portion of lean red meat. If, however, your meat comes as a large thick steak or in the form of mince or sausages, chicken will have less fat. Red meat should be eaten in much smaller and leaner portions than is usual; chicken should also have its fat removed.

Meats can be either very lean or quite fatty. The meats with the lowest fat level are veal, new-fashioned pork (pork fillet, port schnitzel or butterfly steaks), rump, topside or fillet steak, and leg of lamb or lamb leg chops. Remove all fat from meat before cooking it. Once the fat has turned crisp and golden brown, it will be far more irresistible than the cold hard white lump on the raw meat. Marbled fat is much more difficult to remove from any kind of meat; avoid such meats. A small fillet steak with all visible fat removed can fit into a healthy diet. Large T-bones with fat marbled through and a thick edge of fat are likely to increase blood cholesterol levels.

Minced steak presents problems for even the better-quality mince may have a high-fat content. Minced topside steak generally costs less than straight topside and it is unlikely that a butcher will go to the trouble of mincing steak and charge you less for his efforts unless trimmings can be used. The leanest mince comes from fat-trimmed steak which you mince yourself (or have the butcher do it for you).

Cooking

A major problem with very lean meat is that some type of fat is often added during cooking. There is little point in selecting a low-fat veal steak if you then crumb and fry it. Similarly, a piece of fish loses its nutritional virtues if it is battered, fried and served with fat-soaked chips.

Not all meats are suitable for grilling. Steak, chops and fish grill well, but pork or veal can emerge from the griller resembling shoe leather.

You can cook without adding fats. Barbequing or baking foil-wrapped foods seals in all the flavour and produces a succulent sensation in the finished product. For fish, chicken, turkey, veal, pork fillet or a lamb leg chop, take a square of foil for each serve, place the fish or meat in the centre and top with suitable herbs, shallots, celery, sliced mushrooms, lemon or orange slices or some type of fruit. Moisten with about two teaspoons of lemon juice, brandy or wine, and fold foil to make an enclosed parcel. The parcels can be refrigerated until required and then baked or cooked on a barbeque plate. Fish takes about 20 minutes. Meats take anything from 20 to 50 minutes, depending on the cut and size of the portion. There is   183 no washing up as the foil is simply discarded. Baking paper can be used in the same way in the microwave.

The same principle can be used with filo pastry. This has no added fat and can be used without brushing with oil or butter. It is effective in keeping the flavour and juiciness in fish or meat. Simply place each portion on one or two sheets of pastry, top with herbs and vegetables, wrap up and bake in a moderately low oven. The filo goes very crisp and the food being cooked retains its moisture. You can also use two sheets of filo and brush some yoghurt between them. This produces a more pastry-like result with crisp edges.

You can make casseroles and pasta or rice dishes without adding fat. If meat needs to be browned, cut off all fat and brown on a pan-liner in your frying pan or electric frypan or use a non-stick pan. Make your casserole using meat, fish or chicken and add spices, herbs, vegetables, stock, wine or water. Add little water and there will be no need to use thickening. Wine used in cooking contributes flavour, but almost no kilojoules since the alcohol evaporates with heat.

When roasting meat (for example, a lean piece of beef, a leg of lamb or a chicken), remove all fat, rub with mustard or appropriate herbs and spices and place on a rack above a dish containing a little water. The food can also be placed in a roasting pan with a little water, tomato puree, stock or wine. As the liquid evaporates during cooking, add a little more but do not have the meat stewing in a large quantity of water or it will be stringy. The water keeps enough moisture in the oven to prevent the food from drying out. When making sauce or gravy, remove the meat or chicken and keep warm. Add stock, water, wine or fruit juice to the pan drippings and stir well to dissolve any crusty parts. Heat gently until it is boiling and is reduced to a slightly thickened consistency.

With chicken and turkey, lift up the skin and remove any fat. Replace skin and leave on bird while roasting. To reduce fat further, do not eat the skin.

If you are roasting a piece of pork and you love crackling, remove the skin and the adjoining fat layer, scrape off the fat and replace the thin skin over the meat. Rub with dry mustard and garlic for a crisp crackle with only a fraction of the fat of the original piece of meat.

Dinner for those who need to reduce blood fats

Choose lots of vegetables, try to have legumes sometimes, include fish or other seafoods (not cooked in fat), or look for the leanest meats such as turkey fillets, chicken breast, pork fillet, veal or small portions of very lean red meat. Avoid using fats in cooking. Foods such as pasta, potatoes, rice, wheat or any other grain are fine as long as they are not served with fatty sauces.

For dessert, keep to fresh fruits, fruit salad, baked fruits, or recipes made without butter, margarine or cream.

Dinner for those who need to reduce weight

Eat as many vegetables as you like (no one ever grew fat on any kind of vegetables unless they were doused with some type of fat). Try to have fish often as it has far fewer kilojoules than meats. Turkey, chicken breast, new-fashioned pork and veal are also lower in kilojoules than red meats. However, you do not need to avoid red meats entirely. Small portions of lean red meat are a valuable source of iron.

For dessert, have fresh or baked fruits or skip dessert altogether. Some low-kilojoule foods may be useful, for example, low-kilojoule jellies, toppings and low-fat icecream (occasionally).

Dinner for those who must avoid salt

No salt should be used in cooking or serving of foods and avoid stock and sauce mixes (except low-salt varieties), salad dressings and foods canned with salt. Many canned foods are now available in unsalted versions and these are quite suitable.

To make up for the lack of salt, try to make liberal use of herbs and spices. Lemon juice also helps bring out the flavour in many dishes. Try to eat vegetables which have been steamed or microwaved so that more of their flavour is preserved. It can be difficult to make tasty soups without salt. The use of herbs and spices and a good strong stock, made by boiling meat or chicken bones in water, can help overcome the lack of flavour.

Dinner for athletes

Your evening meal needs to contain more of the important carbohydrates. Include pasta, rice, potatoes, cracked wheat, legumes and vegetables as often as possible. Fish, poultry or lean meat can also feature, but should not take the place of the carbohydrates. Add bread or rolls if possible.

Desserts can include fruit, yoghurt, icecream (occasionally) or fruit crumbles.

EATING OUT

There are many restaurants which serve foods that fit easily into a healthy diet. Most, however, use some type of fat in their cooking. If you are only going to eat out every month or so, you only need to make a sensible choice from the menu, avoiding obviously buttery, creamy or fried foods and rich sauces and desserts.

185

For those whose work or lifestyle involves frequent dining in restaurants, a more careful choice is needed. Take care to avoid the 'extras' such as butter with your bread, chips with your meal, chocolates and cream with your coffee. If you find it difficult to resist such temptations, you can either ask for such items to be removed (for example, ask for the butter to be removed from the table or request a meal without chips) or you can take the superlative approach in which you decide only to eat a food if its quality is superb. Decline the mundane chocolates, the standard chips and anything else which is ordinary. Ask yourself whether these foods are worth the kilojoules and fat. This method wipes out about 95 per cent of the extra offerings, since most are really quite ordinary and will be available any time you want them. You can eat and enjoy the remaining few superb examples since they will be an occasional treat rather than a regular part of your eating pattern.

The following suggestions are offered as a simple guide:

Entrees

Soups can be a good choice, as long as they are not thick with heavy cream. Asian-style soups are usually suitable with the exception of those containing fried wontons.

Oysters (natural) are rich in minerals, have almost no fat and are very low in kilojoules and make an ideal entree if you are watching your weight or blood cholesterol.

Seafoods such as prawns, calamari, mussels, crab, lobster and octopus are all low in fat, but are often served fried or in a cream or mayonnaise dressing. Without added fat, they are a great selection.

Salads and vegetables (such as stuffed mushrooms) are a healthy choice as long as they are not drowned in butter or dressing. Ask for dressings to be served separately so that you can use a small portion or avoid them altogether.

Fruits such as melon, with ham or smoked salmon are another low-fat choice. Other exotic fruits are also suitable.

Main courses

You can always avoid large servings by choosing another entree for your main course. Or choose:

Fish, or another seafood, served grilled or poached. You will need to ask for your selection to be served without added butter or oil. Seafood casseroles, bouillabaisse, poached or baked fish are also suitable. Beware of the rich sauces which often accompany such dishes.

Turkey, chicken breast, pork fillet, venison, rabbit, hare, pheasant or any other type of game will have begun its life in the restaurant with very little fat. The final fat content will depend on the way it is cooked and the richness of the accompanying sauce. Fruit- or vegetable-based sauces are usually a good choice. If the sauce is rich, ask for only a very small portion of it to be served.

Red meats will vary according to the establishment where you are eating. In many parts of Australia, steaks are served in 300 to 400-gram portions, an amount which does not fit in with a diet for peak performance. If it appears that large portions are being served, skip the red meat and make another choice. If a red meat choice is unavoidable, try to have a fillet steak and eat only a moderate portion.

Vegetables and/or *salads* also start out with loads of nutrients and no fat. On their way through the restaurant kitchen, many acquire a heavy dose of butter, oil or cream. Ask for steamed vegetables and salads with the dressing served separately. If that is not possible, there is generally less fat in vegetables than in salads.

Bread or rolls are increasingly being replaced with garlic or herb bread, both heavy with butter. Many people regard this as a culinary disaster since bread is meant to offer a respite from the richer flavours of other foods rather than adding a heap of fat. Avoid them and ask for plain bread or rolls instead. Copy the Greeks, Italians, French and Spaniards and skip the butter. In most countries, you would always be served bread, but never butter.

Alcoholic drinks can be the downfall of those who eat out frequently. There is no harm in one or two drinks, but greater quantities hold no joy for your body. Decide which type of alcohol you prefer: a pre-dinner drink, wine with your meal or an after-dinner liqueur. Try to have non-alcoholic drinks the rest of the time. Many people make the mistake of ordering multiple orange juices in place of alcoholic drinks. They may save you from the effects of the alcohol, but are a disaster for those who gain weight easily. A glass of orange juice has the same kilojoules as two slices of bread. Try iced water, mineral or soda water instead.

Desserts have become less popular these days and many people skip them. If you do decide to have dessert, and fresh fruit is available, you cannot make a better choice. A big rich dessert will generally have heaps of fat and sugar. Keep them for special occasions.

Cheeses are too rich in fat to be eaten after a large meal. It makes better nutritional sense to eat cheese with bread, fruit and salad for a meal such as lunch rather than using it as a separate course at dinner. If a cheese platter is unavoidable, your only hope is to take tiny slivers instead of large chunks.

Restaurant guide

Cajun

One of the latest trends in foods, cajun cooking can range from quite healthy food to enormous plates of fatty meats. The spices themselves and the fiery charcoal cooking do not add fat, but servings tend to be large. Try to share portions if possible. Choose seafood dishes, chowders, gumbo (a hearty spicy soup), rice-based creole dishes and any modest serves of charcoal grilled meats. Avoid the enormous plates of ribs unless you are sharing with friends. It will take some days of sober eating to make up for indulging in rich sundaes, pies and other desserts.

Chinese

In China, most foods fit the healthy guidelines. Their translation into Western cuisine often means large quantities of added fat. Choose vegetable, rice, noodle, tofu, seafood, chicken, pork or beef dishes, but avoid anything which has been dipped in batter and/or deep fried. Select boiled rice rather than fried.

French

Choose bouillon, vegetable or seafood soups (without cream), any seafoods (not fried or in rich sauces), main courses as listed on pp 186–7 and fruit for dessert. In France, problems are solved by the small size of the portions and the limited use of meat.

German

Follow the general principles listed for eating out. Try to avoid fatty pork and the excellent, but high-fat, sausages. Potatoes, cabbage, and any other vegetables are good choices. Desserts are often so rich that it will take days of healthy eating to make up for one portion.

Greek

Greek food tends to have loads of olive oil — a healthy product, but best eaten in small quantities. Avoid fried pastry offerings and go for stuffed vine or cabbage leaves, stuffed vegetables, seafoods, spinach dishes, Greek salads (ask for the dressing to be served separately) and souvlaki. Eat the bread, but avoid the pastry desserts.

Indian

Rice and curries are suitable foods. However, some curries begin with a lot of ghee (clarified butter) which can raise the fat content.

In India, vegetable curries and lentils and various legumes predominate and supply dietary fibre and complex carbohydrate. Westerners have a tendency to order mainly meat varieties. Choose some vegetable and seafood curries. Avoid eating too many samosas and other deep-fried foods.

Indonesian

The rice and vegetable dishes are suitable. Sate poultry and meats are generally very lean although the accompanying sauces may be quite oily. Avoid eating too many dishes cooked in coconut cream as it is high in fat.

Italian

Again there is a problem not with the basic ingredients but with the quantity of oil, butter and cream used. Choose seafoods (grilled if possible), pasta with sauces of seafood or vegetables (mushrooms, onion, capsicum, tomatoes), osso bucco (casseroled veal shank), or grilled liver. Most veal dishes are fried and many have added cheese, giving a high total fat content. Parmesan cheese is usually used sparingly in keeping with its strong flavour and presents few problems. Gelato is a low-fat (but high-sugar) dessert.

Japanese

Sushi, sashimi and most other dishes are entirely suitable. Avoid tempura and any other battered or fried foods. In general, the Japanese diet is very healthy and is one of the major reasons why the Japanese live longer than any other race and are almost never overweight.

Lebanese

Many of the foods are great and feature various vegetables. The major problem is the large quantity of olive oil which covers so many dishes. Olive oil is probably the best oil to eat, but too much of any type of fat is undesirable. Try to ask for dishes which have little oil. Eat plenty of the excellent Lebanese bread. Those who are overweight or trying to avoid too much fat should skip the desserts which are heavy with butter, sugar and nuts.

Malaysian

Eat plenty of rice and try some vegetable dishes. Most of the foods are fine and only cause problems when eaten in large quantities.

Mexican

A difficult problem to overcome in many Mexican restaurants is the gigantic size of the portions. Tacos, tortillas and enchilladas are fine and the use of beans is excellent, but you will need to avoid the heavy-handed approach with cheese, meat and sour cream.

Spanish

As with Greek and Italian food, the Spanish make great use of olive oil. In Spain, this is virtually the only form of fat used and the total fat content of the diet is not high. In other countries, however, the oil is added to the fat in meats and many other foods. Try to choose rice dishes, such as paella, seafoods, chicken and various types of vegetables. Try to avoid fats for the next couple of days.

Thai

Again, most foods are fine with the exception of items which have been deep fried. Choose plenty of vegetable dishes and enjoy the boiled rice.

Vegetarian

In theory, vegetarian food can be excellent with loads of vegetables, legumes and fruits. Many vegetarian restaurants feature such healthy choices. Others make up for the lack of meat by heaping on the butter, cheese, cream and other sources of fat. Choose carefully to avoid too much fat.

Vietnamese

As with other Asian cuisines, Vietnamese foods feature vegetables, rice, seafoods, chicken and lean meats. Soups make a good choice and the only things to avoid are the deep-fried foods.

Appendixes

FOR those who are interested in finer details, the following tables set out the approximate levels of various nutrients for particular degrees of body weight and physical activity.

Appendix 1a

HOW MUCH FAT?

The table below indicates the maximum amount of fat appropriate for different levels of physical activity. Once you have determined the desirable level of fat, check out the table of fat values to see that you do not exceed your daily limit. If you eat less than these quantities of fat, so much the better.

Physical activity	approx. kilojoule intake	maximum fat (grams)
Very active (e.g. run 10km/day) Lean	14 500 (3500 cals)	75–100
Moderately active (e.g. run 5km/day) Lean	12 500 (3000 cals)	65–85
Moderately active (e.g. run 5km/day) Need to lose weight	10 000 (2400 cals)	55–65
Some activity (e.g. walk 3km/day) Lean	10 000 (2400 cals)	55–70
Some activity (e.g. walk 3km/day) Need to lose weight	7500 (1800 cals)	40–45
Little activity Lean	7500 (1800 cals)	40–45
Little activity Need to lose weight	6500 (1500 cals)	35–40

191

The kilojoule requirements given on the previous page are approximate and are intended only as a guide to appropriate fat levels to include in the daily diet. The average woman would need to reduce the levels by about 20 per cent to account for a smaller body size. Large-framed women may need no reduction.

Appendix 1b

HOW MUCH SUGAR?

The table below indicates an appropriate amount of sugar for different levels of physical activity. Once you have found your ideal level of sugar, check out the table of sugar values for different foods. If you would like to eat less sugar than is listed below, rest assured that you will not be doing your body the slightest harm.

Physical activity	approx. kilojoule intake	sugar intake (grams)
Very active (e.g. run 10km/day) Lean	14 500 (3500 cals) or more	80–90
Moderately active (e.g. run 5km/day) Lean	12 500 (3000 cals)	55–60
Moderately active (e.g. run 5km/day) Need to lose weight	10 000 (2400 cals)	0–45
Some activity (e.g. walk 3km/day) Lean	10 000 (2400 cals)	30–60
Some activity (e.g. walk 3km/day) Need to lose weight	7500 (1800 cals)	0–35
Little activity Lean	7500 (1800 cals)	25–45
Little activity Need to lose weight	6500 (1500 cals)	0–20

The kilojoule requirements given above are approximate and are intended only as a guide. The average woman may need to reduce the levels by about 20 per cent to account for a smaller body size. Tall, large-framed women may need no reduction.

HOW MUCH TOTAL CARBOHYDRATE?

Physical activity	approx. kilojoule intake	minimum carbohydrate* (grams)
Very active (e.g. run 10km/day) Lean	14 500 (3500 cals) or more	525
Moderately active (e.g. run 5km/day) Lean	12 500 (3000 cals)	450
Moderately active (e.g. run 5km/day) Need to lose weight	10 000 (2400 cals)	360
Some activity (e.g. walk 3km/day) Lean	10 000 (2400 cals)	360
Some activity (e.g. walk 3km/day) Need to lose weight	7500 (1800 cals)	270
Little activity Lean	7500 (1800 cals)	270
Little activity Need to lose weight	6500 (1500 cals)	225

*The ideal forms of carbohydrate are from complex carbohydrates (see page 60), and from fruits or milk (see pp 60–1). Sugar can make up a small portion of this carbohydrate if desired, but should not be greater than the amounts listed in Appendix 1b

The kilojoule requirements given are approximate and are intended only as a guide to appropriate levels of carbohydrates to include in the daily diet. The average woman would need to reduce the levels by about 20 per cent to account for a smaller body size. Large-framed women may need no reduction.

Appendix 1d

HOW MUCH PROTEIN?

Physical activity	approx. kilojoule intake	protein (grams)
Very active (e.g. run 10km/day) Lean	14 500 (3500 cals)	90–130
Moderately active (e.g. run 5km/day) Lean	12 500 (3000 cals)	75–110

Physical activity	approx. kilojoule intake	protein (grams)
Moderately active (e.g. run 5km/day) Need to lose weight	10 000 (2400 cals)	60–90
Some activity (e.g. walk 3km/day) Lean	10 000 (2400 cals)	60–90
Some activity (e.g. walk 3km/day) Need to lose weight	7500 (1800 cals)	45–70
Little activity Lean	7500 (1800 cals)	45–70
Little activity Need to lose weight	6500 (1500 cals)	40–55

The kilojoule requirements given above are approximate and are intended only as a guide to appropriate protein levels to include in the daily diet. The average woman would need to reduce the levels by about 20 per cent to account for a smaller body size. Large-framed women may need no reduction. See Table 8.1 for the quantities of protein in particular foods.

Appendix 1e

HEALTHY MUESLI

500g rolled oats
1/4 cup sesame seeds
1/2 cup coconut flakes
250g rolled rye or barley flakes* (or use a mixture)
1 cup oat bran
1 cup wheatgerm
1 cup dried fruit medley (apricots, apples, pears, sultanas)
1 cup sultanas
1/2 cup pepitas*
1 cup sunflower seeds
1/2 cup roasted buckwheat*

Toast oats by placing them on a flat, ungreased oven tray in a moderate oven for 5 to 10 minutes, stirring occasionally until oats brown (some oats take longer than others). Toast sesame seeds and coconut by the same method. While toasted ingredients are cooling, mix remaining ingredients together. Add cooled oats, seeds and coconut.
Makes 30 serves of 50 grams each.

*Available from health food stores

HERB AND SPICE GUIDE

Herb	*Uses*
Basil	With tomatoes, in spaghetti sauces, with mushrooms, cream or cottage cheese, peas or carrots, lamb or venison.
Bay leaves	With tomatoes, artichokes, mushrooms, lamb casseroles, marinades, pickles.
Cardamom	Fruits, yoghurt, curries, pork, cakes.
Chervil	Looks like parsley, mild anise flavour; use in soups, sauces, salads, egg dishes, cream or cottage cheese, poultry, fish.
Chives	Mild onion flavour goes with soups, sandwiches, salads, egg dishes, fish, poultry, pork or other meats, potatoes, vegetables.
Cinnamon	As well as use on toast and in desserts, try it with grapefruit, spiced nuts, popcorn, chicken, pork, ham or turkey.
Cloves	For use in cakes and desserts and goes well with oranges, chicken, yoghurt and fruit salad.
Coriander	Goes well with Asian dishes and in salads, soups, curries, rice.
Dill	Excellent in salads, with potatoes, egg dishes, fish or other seafood, rice or pasta.
Fennel	Similar to dill but either foliage or bulb can be used. Same uses as dill.
Ginger	Used in cakes, with chicken, fish, poultry, pork, venison, carrots, with cottage or cream cheese.
Horseradish	Good with beef, pork, fish and in salads, soups or sauces.
Lemon grass	Slice very finely and add to rice, Asian style dishes, chicken, fish.

195

Herb	Uses
Lemon thyme	Delicate flavour goes well with fish, other seafoods, chicken, pork, salads, sandwiches, vegetables such as potatoes, pumpkin, carrots, cauliflower.
Marjoram	Excellent with Mediterranean style dishes including fish, chicken, beef, eggs, soups, salads, in marinades, sliced on sandwiches, or with cauliflower, peas or tomatoes.
Mint	Excellent with lamb or in salads, with potatoes, pineapple, cracked wheat salad, rice, fruit salad.
Oregano	The wild form of marjoram; uses similar to marjoram.
Paprika	As a garnish for eggs, cottage or cream cheese, salads, chicken or potatoes or use in soups, sauces casseroles, pasta.
Parsley	In salads, sandwiches, soups, sauces, on top of pasta, rice, chicken, fish or meats, almost any vegetables, or with eggs.
Poppy seeds	Add flavour to breads, potatoes, pasta or rice dishes.
Rosemary	Good with lamb, chicken or fish, vegetables, especially eggplant, tomatoes, zucchini, onions, bean dishes, pasta or rice.
Sage	Flavours lamb, pork, poultry, bean dishes, cheese and egg dishes, stuffings, salads, pasta sauces.
Savoury	Excellent with beans or dried peas, vegetables such as zucchini, tomatoes, mushrooms, eggplant, pumpkin.
Sorrel	Slightly bitter, lemon flavour goes well in sauces for fish, chicken or in salads, soups, egg dishes, pasta or potatoes.
Tarragon	Delicate flavour goes well with eggs, potatoes, fish and other seafoods, chicken, turkey, in salad dressings, on salads or with rice or pasta.
Thyme	Good with liver, lamb, chicken, turkey, pork, veal, venison, tomatoes, onions, omelettes, herbed breads, pasta dishes.

Appendix 1g RECOMMENDED DAILY AMOUNTS OF FOOD ENERGY AND SOME NUTRIENTS FOR POPULATION GROUPS IN THE UK

Age range [a] (years)	Occupational category	Energy [b] MJ	Energy [b] Kcal	Protein [c] g	Thiamin mg	Riboflavin mg	Nicotinic acid equivalents mg [d]	Ascorbic acid mg	Vitamin A retinol equivalents µg [e]	Vitamin D [f] cholecalciferol µg	Calcium [l] mg	Iron mg
BOYS under 1					0.3	0.4	5	20	450	7.5	600	6
2		5.75	1400	35	0.6	0.7	8	20	300	10	600	7
5–6		7.25	1740	43	0.7	0.9	10	20	300	[f]	600	10
9–11		9.5	2280	57	0.9	1.2	14	25	575	[f]	700	12 [h]
15–17		12.0	2880	72	1.2	1.7	19	30	750	[f]	600	12 [h]
GIRLS under 1					0.3	0.4	5	20	450	7.5	600	6
2		5.5	1300	32	0.5	0.7	8	20	300	10	600	7
5–6		7.0	1680	42	0.7	0.9	10	20	300	[f]	600	10
9–11		8.5	2050	51	0.8	1.2	14	25	575	[f]	700	12 [h]
15–17		9.0	2150	53	0.9	1.7	19	30	750	[f]	600	12 [h]
MEN 18–34	Sedentary	10.5	2510	63	1.0	1.6	18	30	750	[f]	500	10
	Moderately active	12.0	2900	72	1.2	1.6	18	30	750	[f]	500	10
	Very active	14.0	3350	84	1.3	1.6	18	30	750	[f]	500	10
35–64	Sedentary	10.0	2400	60	1.0	1.6	18	30	750	[f]	500	10
	Moderately active	11.5	2750	69	1.1	1.6	18	30	750	[f]	500	10
	Very active	14.0	3350	84	1.3	1.6	18	30	750	[f]	500	10
65–74	Assuming a	10.0	2400	60	1.0	1.6	18	30	750	[f]	500	10
75+	sedentary life	9.0	2150	54	0.9	1.6	18	30	750	[f]	500	10
WOMEN 18–54	Most occupations	9.0	2150	54	0.9	1.3	15	30	750	[f]	500	12 [h]
	Very active	10.5	2500	62	1.0	1.3	15	30	750	[f]	500	12 [h]
55–74	Assuming a	8.0	1900	47	0.8	1.3	15	30	750	[f]	500	10
75+	sedentary life	7.0	1680	42	0.7	1.3	15	30	750	[f]	500	10
Pregnancy		10.0	2400	60	1.0	1.6	18	60	750	10	1200 [g]	13
Lactation		11.5	2750	69	1.1	1.8	21	60	1200	10	1200	15

Notes:

(a) Since the recommendations are average amounts, the figures for each age range represent the amounts recommended at the middle of the range. Within each age range, younger children will need less, and older children more, than the amount recommended.

(b) Megajoules (10^6 joules) Calculated from the relation 1 kilocalorie = 4,184 kilojoules, that is to say, 1 megajoule = 240 kilocalories.

(c) Recommended amounts have been calculated as 10% of the recommendations for energy.

(d) 1 nicotinic acid equivalent = 1 mg available nicotinic acid or 60 mg tryptophan.

(e) 1 retinol = 1 µg retinol or 6 µg β carotene or 12 µg other biologically active carotenoids.

(f) No dietary sources may be necessary for children and adults who are sufficiently exposed to sunlight, but during the winter children and adolescents should receive 10 µg (400 i.u.) daily by supplementation. Adults with inadequate exposure to sunlight, for example those who are housebound, may also need a supplement of 10 µg daily.

(g) For the third trimester only.

(h) This intake may not be sufficient for 10% of girls and women with large menstrual losses.

Source: HMSO

Appendix 1h

HEALTHY WEIGHT RANGE

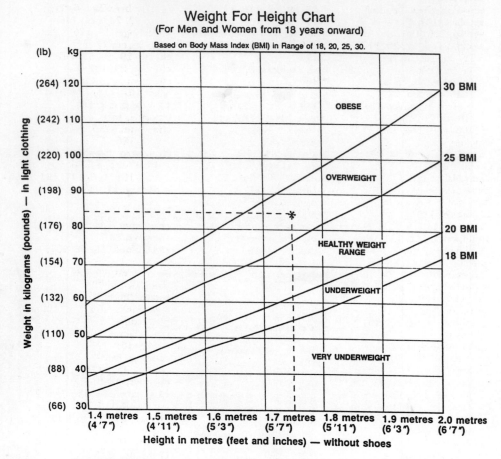

Weight For Height Chart
(For Men and Women from 18 years onward)
Based on Body Mass Index (BMI) in Range of 18, 20, 25, 30.

Reproduced with the permission of the Australian Nutrition Foundation Inc.

Index

acesulfame K, 47
acetic acid, 66
advertising, 2
aerobic activity, 58, 157
aerobics, 167
ageing, 126, 130
alcohol, 7–8, 14, 20, 21, 75–85, 164; absorption, 77–9, 85; and dehydration, 78–9; concentration, 77–8; content in drinks, 84–5; effects, 77–9, 80, 81, 106, 110, 115, 132, 133
amines, 79
amino acids, 56, 87, 88, 90, 160
amygdalin, 162
anaemia, 98–9, 132, 134
anaerobic activity, 58, 157
anorexia, 113
antacids, 116
antibiotics, 132, 135
antioxidant, 130
aphrodisiacs, 81, 83–4
appetite, 70, 154
apricot kernels, 162, 163
arginine, 160
arthritis, 15, 144
artificial sweeteners, 40, 46–7
ascorbic acid: see vitamin C
aspartame, 47
aspirin, 98, 127
athletes, 31, 33, 59, 90, 98, 99, 105, 113, 126, 156–172, 178, 181, 185; and sugar, 47–8, 50; water losses, 55
avidin, 135
avocados, 17, 18, 24

bacteria, 29–30, 69, 94, 119, 131, 132, 135
bananas, 53
beans, 90; see also legumes
beansprouts, 21
bee pollen, 163
beer, 7, 76, 80
beer gut, 141, 142
behaviour: and alcohol, 78; and diet, 42
bile acids, 69
bile salts, 20
binge eating, 113

bioflavenoids, 162
blood pressure, 79, 80, 81, 93, 116, 129; high, 7, 28, 29, 32, 115, 141, 143; low, 29
blood sugar, 10, 58, 69–70, 139, 157–8, 168, 170, 179
body builders, 87, 89, 159, 160
body shape, 141–3, 145, 154
bones, 104–5, 115, 144, 163
bowel, 65–8
brain, 80, 81, 170
bran, 21, 64, 66, 102, 111
bread, 33, 53, 90, 102, 146, 179, 187; consumption, 8, 9
breakfast, 151, 174, 175–9
breast milk, 44, 111, 132
breast: fat tissue and cancer, 143–4
butter, 16
butyric acid, 66

caffeine, 83, 106, 165
Cajun meals, 188
calcium, 29, 88, 94, 104–9, 129, 130, 163; in foods, 108–9; supplements, 108
cancer, 16, 17, 81, 93, 123, 125, 126, 130, 133, 162; bowel, 66, 68–9, 80, 143–4; hormone dependent, 143–4; oesophagus, 80; stomach, 30
canned foods, 185
carbohyrate, 48, 53–61, 137, 145, 146, 157–8, 161, 168–9 complex, 3, 4, 8–10, 25, 52–62, 70, 91, 140, 146, 148, 170, 171, 181; digestion of, 55–6; in foods, 60–1; level in diet, 137, 140; requirements, Appendix 1c; simple, 59; sugar, 6, 48
carbohydrate loading, 139, 168–170
carnitine, 162

carob bars, 4
carotene, 122–4
cellulose, 65, 66
cereals: breakfast, 6, 11, 45, 50, 72, 124, 176; porridge, 11, 176
champagne, 77
cheese, 29–30, 33, 187
chicken, 23, 182–3
children: fat, 141; diet, 42, 87, 102, 111, 174–5
Chinese meals, 188
chloride, 163
chocolate, 5, 15, 24, 165, 171, 186
cholesterol: blood, 10, 15, 16, 17–21, 54, 66, 69, 125, 134, 135, 177, 183; dietary, 17, 18–19, 20–1, 177
choline, 21;
chromium, 45
cirrhosis, 80
clots, blood, 18, 22, 131, 132
coconut oil, 15, 18
cod liver oil, 129
coffee, 83, 164
cola drinks, 165
confectionery, 43
constipation, 10, 64, 66–8, 103, 163
cooking, 183–4
copper, 111, 125
corn syrup, 40, 46
Cornflakes, 10, 33
cot death, 133, 135
cramps, 31–2, 156, 158, 164
cricket, 167
croissant, 5, 25
cyanocobalamin: see vitamin B$_{12}$
cyclamate, 46
cycling, 157, 166, 168

dairy products, 15, 18, 24, 148, 172
dehydration, 9, 78–9, 111, 164–5; see also water loss
dextrose, 43
DHA, 16
diabetes, 42–3, 133, 141, 143; diet, 46, 70

199

diarrhoea, 67, 101, 111, 115, 127, 133, 134, 158
dietary fibre, 5, 10–11, 20–1, 23, 63–74, 146; digestion of, 56, 65–6, 67; in foods, 71–3; soluble, 66; types, 65;
Dietary Guidelines, 41
diets: see weight reduction diets
digestion, 55–7
dinner, 153, 174, 181–3
diuretics, 113, 115
diverticulitis, 67
drinks, 164–5; diet, 144; sports, 115, 163, 164; and alcohol, 82–3
drugs: and vitamins, 134

eating habits, 2
eggs, 15, 18, 19, 21, 89, 135, 160, 177
electrolytes, 27
emulsifiers, 21
endurance exercise, 58–9, 70, 88, 94–5, 157, 158, 159, 161, 164, 167–170
energy, 88, 98, 119, 162, 164, 174; see also kilojoules; fuel for, 3–4, 6, 8, 9, 48, 157–160, 165–8; requirements, 12, 157
enzymes, 56, 157
EPA, 16
ethanol, 76
exercise, 3, 12, 54–5, 58–9, 105–106, 138, 140, 142–3, 145, 147, 148–9, 154, 164–9; passive, 144; and sugar, 47–8

fast foods, 15, 18, 28, 32, 181
fasting, 58, 111, 113
fat: body, 4, 9, 12, 14–15, 19, 56, 57, 58, 113, 137, 138, 139, 140–5, 154, 157, 158;
fat cells, 140–1
fat content of foods, 23–4
fatigue, 98, 124, 126, 168, 169
fats, 13–25, 144, 148; animal, 15, 18; digestion of, 55–6; in blood, 19–20, 21–2, 70, 79, 80, 143, 148, 159; in foods,

4–5, 6, 14, 66, 168; monounsaturated, 15, 17; polyunsaturated, 15, 16, 21, 89, 130; requirements, Appendix 1a; saturated, 15, 17, 18, 19, 88, 89; vegetable, 16
fatty acids, 5, 16, 134, 135; as fuel, 58, 157, 158–9, 161, 162, 168; volatile, 66, 69
ferritin, 98, 99, 103
fibre supplements, 67–8
fibre: see dietary fibre
figs, 156
filo pastry, 184
fish oil capsules, 22
fish, 19, 23, 107, 182; fats in, 16, 22, 162
flatulence, 71, 170
fluid, 137–8, 139–140, 164: see also water
folate, 134
food labels, 44–5
football, 167, 169
French meals, 188
fructose, 44, 59, 83
fruit juice, 10, 11, 187
fruit, 2, 4, 10, 11, 12, 23, 25, 35, 44, 53, 65, 69, 73, 115, 116, 122, 124, 127, 150, 175; citrus, 162; dried, 35
fruitarians, 89
fuel, 58–9, 157, 175; see also energy

gallstones, 69, 141, 143
game, 187
gelatine, 89
gels, 65
German meals, 188
glucose polymers, 165
glucose, 43, 47, 55, 56–7, 157–8, 164, 168, 170; in blood, 66, 158; see also blood sugar
glycaemic index, 56
glycerol, 56
glycogen, 3, 10, 12, 47, 48, 56, 57–9, 62, 133, 139, 140, 157–8, 159, 161, 165, 167–9, 176, 179
golden syrup, 45
gout, 133
grazing, 174–5
Greek meals, 188
guar gum, 70

gums, 65

haemoglobin, 98–9, 103, 130, 133, 134
haemorrhoids, 67
hair analysis, 110
hair loss, 124
hair, 135; grey, 134
hangover, 78–9
HDL cholesterol, 19–20
health bars, 45
heart disease, 15, 16, 17, 18, 22, 141, 143
heart muscle, 113
hemicellulose, 65, 66
herb and spice guide: Appendix 1f
honey , 44, 45
hormones: female, 105
hunger, 58, 70, 157
hyperactivity, 42
hypertension: see blood pressure, high

icecream, 4, 24
Indian meals, 188–9
Indonesian meals, 189
insulin, 42, 48, 56, 143, 158, 168
iron, 94, 98–104, 124, 163; deficiency, 99, 103, 111; haem, 101–2; non-haem, 101–2; requirements, 101; sources, 103; supplements, 103–4
irritable bowel syndrome, 67
Italian meals, 189

jam, low kilojoule, 177
Japanese meals, 189
junk foods, 2, 145

kidney function, 27–8
kidney stones, 108, 127, 129
kilojoules, 12, 53, 57, 145–6, 148–9, 174; from alcohol, 7, 8, 57, 77; from carbohydrate, 53, 57, 62; from fat, 4, 5, 14, 15, 17, 23, 57; from protein, 57, 91; from sugar, 6, 41, 42, 43, 44, 48, 51

lactation, 99, 110, 126,

133, 134, 142
lactose, 44, 59, 107
laetrile, 162
laxatives, 10, 67–8, 113, 116
LDL cholesterol, 19–20
Lebanese meals, 189
lecithin, 21
legumes, 21, 53, 66, 69, 70, 71, 146
lignin, 65, 66, 69
linoleic acid, 16
linolenic acid, 16, 162
linseeds, 162
lipoprotein, 19
liqueurs, 76
lunch, 152, 174, 179–81

magnesium, 115–17, 163, 168; in foods, 116–17; requirements, 116
maltose, 44
mannitol, 46
margarine, 15, 16, 24
meals, 174–190
meat, 18, 19, 23, 25, 93, 94, 100, 104, 182–3, 187
meat pies, 4
mega–dose vitamins, 121–2
men: and alcohol, 79–81; and body fat, 81, 141–2; and meat, 99, 156;
menstrual cycle, 8, 14, 82, 99, 105, 138, 142, 163
mercury, 127
metabolism, 137, 140, 148, 149, 151, 166, 174, 175
Mexican meals, 190
microwaves, 127, 128, 133, 182, 184
milk, 59, 104, 107, 108, 160
minerals, 98, 162
molasses, 45
mood, 125
mucilages, 65
muesli, 4, 177; recipe: recipe: Appendix 1e
multi-vitamins, 121, 135
muscles, 87–8, 130, 138, 145, 146, 159–160; energy for, 3, 4, 6, 8, 9, 126, 139, 140, 157–60
mushrooms, 94

nausea, 158, 164

niacin, 133, 161
nitrates, 125
nitrosamines, 80, 125
NutraSweet: see aspartame
nuts, 73

oats, 21, 65, 66, 69, 70, 146, 176, 177
obesity: see overweight
oestrogen, 108, 143
olive oil, 17, 188, 189
omega-3 fatty acids, 16, 22, 23
omega-6 fatty acids, 16
oral contraceptives, 124
ornithine, 160
orotic acid, 162
osteomalacia, 128
osteoporosis, 15, 29, 104–5, 144, 163
overweight, 41, 137–49, 174
oxalic acid, 102, 106, 127
oysters, 102, 111, 186
ozone, 130

palm oil, 15, 18
pangamic acid, 162
pantothenic acid, 134, 163
pasteurisation, 133
peanut butter, 177
peanut oil, 17
pectin, 20–1, 65, 68, 69
phenylalanine, 47
phosphates, 111
phospholipids, 21
phosphorus, 105
physical activity, 2–3, 8, 23, 59, 140, 142, 148–9, 165–8; and salt, 27, 31; and sugar, 6; and water, 27; diet for, 11–12, 54, 155–72
phytic acid, 64, 102, 111
pins and needles, 98
PKU, 47
polysaccharide, 65
potassium, 27, 28, 33, 35, 37, 113–15, 163, 164, 168; in foods, 114; requirements, 113
potato crisps, 33, 54
potatoes, 9, 53, 70, 146
prawns, 19
pre-event meal, 170–1
pre-menstrual syndrome, 133

pregancy, 99, 110, 126, 133, 134, 142; and alcohol, 82
preservatives, 29–30
Pritikin diet, 54, 59
processed foods, 15, 28, 30, 32, 33, 35, 65, 67, 68, 70, 114, 119, 120, 121; salt content, 29–30
processed meats, 25
propionic acid, 66
prostaglandins, 162
protein powders, 90–1, 159, 160
protein, 4, 11, 86–96, 106, 148, 156, 159–60, 168; animal, 88–9; complementary, 89–90; digestion of, 55–6; requirements, 91, Appendix 1d; sources, 91, 92; vegetable, 88–9, 91
pyridoxine: see vitamin B$_6$

restaurant meals, 180, 181, 185–90
retinol: see vitamin A
riboflavin, 133, 161
ricotta cheese, 107
roughage, 64; see also dietary fibre
royal jelly, 163
rum, 39–40, 84
running, 166

saccharin, 46
salad dressing, 182
salmon, 182
salt, 7, 26–37, 106, 138, 164–5, 178, 185; substitutes, 35–6
saponins, 21, 65, 69
sea salt, 35
seafood, 24, 25, 186
selenium, 130
serendipity berry, 46
sesame seeds, 106, 107
shellfish, 19
skin, 119, 124, 125, 129, 133, 134, 135
slimming diets: see weight reduction diets
smoking, 106, 126, 149; and weight gain, 149–153
snacks, 152, 153, 176

Index

sodium, 7, 27–8, 31, 33, 113, 114, 138, 163, 164, 168
soft drinks, 6, 43
sorbitol, 46
soya beans, 107
soyabean protein, 160
Spanish meals, 190
spinach, 102
spirits, 76
sport: and diet, 156–72, 175
sprinting, 157, 166, 169
squash, 166
starches, 53–4; see also carbohydrate, complex
starvation, 139
stock: chicken, 182
stomach, 55–6
stress, 126
stroke, 32, 38–51;
sucrose, 44;
sugar beet, 40;
sugar, 5–6, 21, 56–7, 158, 164, 168, 170; appropriate amounts, Appendix 1b; brown, 45; in foods, 49–50; raw, 45–6
sunlight, 128, 129
supplements: for sport, 156; see also vitamin supplements
sweating, 7, 27, 30, 111, 113, 163, 164;
swimming, 157, 167, 171

take away foods, 180; see also fast foods
tannin, 102
tea, 102, 164
teeth, 40, 41
tennis, 166–7
Thai meals, 190
thiamin, 121, 133, 161
thyroid gland, 131, 133
tocopherols, 129
tofu, 91
tofu icecream, 4
treacle, 45
triathletes, 158
triglycerides, 21–2, 80
tuna, 182
turkey, 23, 25, 182

underweight, 144, 153–4
uric acid, 127

vegan diet, 94, 95–6
Vegemite, 33, 176–7
vegetable oils, 16, 17
vegetable salt, 35
vegetables, 4, 10, 11, 12, 25, 30, 35, 53, 65, 72, 90, 101, 102, 115, 116, 122, 124, 127, 132, 146, 147–8, 181–2, 187; frozen, 128
vegetarian diet, 93–6, 102, 110, 134, 159
vegetarian meals, 190
vitamin A, 122–4, 161
vitamin B, 83, 124–5, 133–5
vitamin B_1 : see thiamin
vitamin B_2 : see riboflavin
vitamin B_3 : see niacin
vitamin B_6, 133, 161
vitamin B_{12}, 94, 134, 161
vitamin B_{13}, 162
vitamin B_{15}, 162
vitamin B_{17}, 162
vitamin B-T, 162
vitamin C, 83, 102, 103, 125–8, 161, 161, 163
vitamin D, 17, 105, 128–9, 131, 161
vitamin E, 17, 119–20, 124, 129–31, 161
vitamin F, 162
vitamin K, 131–2
vitamin P, 162
vitamin supplements, 98, 119, 120–2, 161–2, 172
vitamins, 3, 118–35, 157, 161–2; deficiency, 2, 121; excess, 120, 123–4, 126–7, 129, 131, 132, 133–5; Recommended Daily Intakes, Appendix 1g

walking, 157, 165–6
water, 27–8, 47–8, 55, 68, 138, 156, 164–5, 168; hard, 115; loss, 9, 31, 32, 68, 139, 164–5
weight, 137–54; healthy range, Appendix 1h
weight loss, 9, 57, 58, 136–53
weight reduction diets, 3, 54, 57, 59, 99–100, 177–8, 180, 185, 137–41, 144–8, 151–3

weight training, 87, 160
weight, to gain, 153–4
wheatgerm, 120
wholergrains, 64, 65, 146, 148
wine, 76, 79, 184
women: and alcohol, 78, 81, 82; and calcium, 94, 104–5, 108, 109; and iron, 94, 98, 99, 101, 103; body fat, 14, 105, 141–2, 163

xylitol, 46

zinc, 94, 101, 109–12, 124, 125; in foods, 112; requirements, 110

202